THE GIFT

THE GIFT

*Stroke Survival:
From Recovery to
Thriving. A Spiritual
Awakening -
Embracing
Resilience, Courage,
and Transformation
through the
Law of Attraction*

SIMON KENT

Quantum Twenty One Publishing

For permission requests, contact the publisher at simon.kent@quantumtwentyone.com

Cover art by: Simon Kent & Claire Chapman

Cover image by: Simon Kent

ISBN: 978-1-7393945-4-7

eBook: 978-1-7393945-5-4

Published by: Quantum Twenty One Publishing (Quantum Twenty One Ltd)

Disclaimer

The information contained in this book, titled "The Gift" is based solely on the personal experiences and insights of the author. The author is not a medical professional, and the content presented in this book is not intended to provide medical advice, diagnose medical conditions, or replace professional medical guidance.

The purpose of this book is to share the author's personal journey of survival and recovery from a stroke. The author acknowledges that every individual's experience with stroke is unique, and the recovery process can vary significantly from person to person.

Readers are advised to consult qualified medical professionals, such as physicians, neurologists, therapists, and other healthcare providers, for accurate and personalised medical advice and treatment recommendations. The information presented in this book should not be considered a substitute for professional medical evaluation, diagnosis, or treatment.

The author makes no claims, guarantees, or warranties regarding the effectiveness of any methods, practices, or techniques mentioned in this book for the recovery from stroke. The author disclaims any liability for any loss or damage, whether direct or indirect, that may arise from the use or reliance on the information provided in this book.

Ultimately, the decision to pursue any medical treatment, therapy, or lifestyle changes should be made in consultation with qualified medical professionals who have a comprehensive understanding of the individual's medical history, current condition, and unique needs.

By reading this book, you acknowledge and agree to the terms of this disclaimer.

Please consult a medical professional before making any healthcare decisions or changes to your treatment plan.

Acknowledgements

There are so many people to thank, but first and foremost, my deepest love, thanks and appreciation go to my life partner and fiance, Claire, without whom I might not have recovered quite as well as I have. On many occasions, she knows me better than I know myself and whilst that can be uncomfortable at times, she has always challenged me from a place of love and for my highest good. Thank you, Claire, I love you so much and this book is for you as much as it is for me.

Huge thanks to our blended family of Charlotte, Eva, William and Logan, thanks for helping to "keep it real" guys, and to my eldest daughter Bryony with Jack, thanks for all your love from the other side of the world in Australia, I always feel your love, even from afar. Massive thanks for the support network we have had around Claire and I which has been truly incredible. Very special thanks and a lot of love go to Gemma and Kevin Tullett, Anita and Roger Gough, and The Bowers Family (Lins, Alfie and gang). Unbelievable gratitude goes to all the staff at NHS Oxford University Hospitals John Radcliffe Neurosciences Department, all the staff at NHS Great Western Hospitals Falcon Ward, Swindon (Acute

Stroke Unit), all the staff of NHS Wiltshire Integrated Neurology and Stroke Service (The ESD Team especially Lara, Kate, Sue & Alice), with special mentions for Amy, Anton and the physio team, and Kris (Wiltshire NHS Ambulance Service), Dr Andrew Kirtley (Clinical Psychologist). Thank you to RWBRFC (Royal Wootton Bassett Rugby Football Club), my brother, sister and sister-in-law, Phil, Jo and Pen Kent (thank you Phil for those early inspirational conversations) and thanks to Tim Mills and John Noctor for the contract work, great conversations and for believing in me. Thank you, Nicky Marshall and Sue Stone for the support, encouragement and advice for the book(s). Thank you to Donna, Craig Ross, and team members for your kindness and BTC-based financial help.

To the stroke survivor support groups and charities Different Strokes and A Stroke of Luck, you are rock stars that provide a valuable service and community to those whose lives have been dramatically altered by Stroke; keep up the great work.

Thanks go out to all my online friends and connections who have given so much love and support on my social media posts during my recovery that helped support the idea of the creation of this and other books. Your support spurred me on to get this done.

With the online world in mind, I also thank everyone who gave me feedback on the cover design, specifically Simone Jo Moore, Julie Cleary and Alicia Ng all of whose specific feedback led to alterations in my design.

My thanks go to all those who sent me personal messages of support and care in those early days of recovery, especially Barclay Rae, I think you may have been the first to call me in the hospital; I won't forget that, and Mats Stadin Gomf; your generosity with the music will also, never be forgotten.

Three people have now sadly passed but they are within my mind often. Firstly, my mother, Lorna, who passed on the same day that I received the very first physical copy of this book, the synchronicity of which carries great meaning for me. Mum, my understanding of you runs profound, and I have cherished memories of conversations that bring warmth to my heart. Secondly, my father, Richard Kent, whose passing in March 2022 occurred just 6 months after my stroke. Dad, I now grasp the lessons and wisdom you imparted in your lifetime. Your wisdom left a mark on my heart and for that, I am eternally grateful. Mum and Dad, my love for you both remains forever unwavering. Thirdly, the late, great Leslie Fiegler, whom I got to know in 2022 as a student of some of his outstanding work, for which, I am eternally grateful.

Finally, I have the deepest love and gratitude for rediscovering the universal God inside of myself and all others, without which none of my recovery would have happened at all.

Note to readers

First and foremost, I want to express my heartfelt gratitude for your commitment to reading this book. Your interest in my story truly means the world to me, and I genuinely hope that you not only enjoy it but also gain profound insights from my experience.

The book commences with my personal narrative detailing the unfolding of the stroke's events. In the initial six months of my recovery, I began crafting social media posts, which subsequently served as the foundation for the rest of the story. These posts are seamlessly woven into each chapter, commencing with Chapter 9, aptly titled "September 23, 2021: F..K That Hurts!"

Subsequently, each post is accompanied by an additional narrative crafted approximately 3-6 months after the original social media entry. These narratives serve to further delve into the essence of the initial post, offering a profound catharsis and spiritual evolution. Following this narrative is a succinct paragraph or even a single sentence, encapsulating a message I've termed a "transformation key." The entirety of these transformation keys is compiled in another book I've titled "The Transformation Keys."

"The Transformation Keys" is accessible in both physical and online formats. While "The Gift" chronicles my personal journey and offers self-help as a result of that journey, "The Transformation Keys" is designed specifically as a self-help book with broad appeal, offering guidance for individuals navigating personal transformations across any aspect of life. In many ways, the two books make a perfect partnership, as one was created directly from the other.

Contents

HOME - THE ANNEX

HOME - FAMILY HOME

Contents ~ xvii

Introduction

This is a story about many things besides brain haemorrhage (haemorrhagic stroke) and my journey of recovery. It is also a story about resilience, humility, perseverance, surrender, determination, courage, acceptance, forgiveness and grace. But then it's also about perspective and the transformation of a human being (aka me) as a result of being forced to stop by an event that no one could have predicted or controlled. It's a story of my profound spiritual awakening, or perhaps I should say re-awakening, and how the Universal Law of Attraction played out in my recovery. There are many lessons within this book; Lessons for me and, I hope, lessons for you as well.

Let's start by explaining what a haemorrhagic stroke is. Before my experience of a brain haemorrhage, I had no idea that such an event was even classified as a type of stroke. There are essentially three types of stroke, Ischaemic stroke, Haemorrhagic stroke and Transient ischaemic attack (TIA). An Ischaemic stroke is the most common type of stroke and is caused by a blockage cutting off the blood supply to the brain. A haemorrhagic stroke is caused by bleeding in or around the brain. A transient ischaemic attack (TIA) is also known as a mini-stroke. It is the same as a stroke, except the symptoms typically only last for a short amount of time because the blockage that stops the blood supply from reaching the brain is temporary (hence transient).

I experienced a haemorrhagic stroke. According to The Stroke Association website, 15% of strokes are haemorrhagic. Within this category, there are two types, ICH and SAH. I experienced an ICH. An ICH means Intracerebral haemorrhage which is when blood leaks out of a blood vessel into the brain tissue. Around 66% of haemorrhagic strokes are ICH. There can be numerous causes and in my case, it was eventually concluded that the cause was high blood pressure (hypertension). The ICH I experienced was called a Posterior ICH, which means it occurred in the back of the brain, specifically the cerebellum area of my brain. Upon investigation and following numerous tests, there was no conclusive medical reason for my high blood pressure, so I have had to draw my own conclusions about probable causes.

When any type of stroke occurs it permanently damages the affected brain tissue, and the brain has to then create new neurology to replace the damaged brain tissue. Also, having any form of brain damage severely impacts the entire brain, not just the immediate area (i.e. Cerebellum in my case). I once read that neurology within the brain can be compared to a global network (e.g. the World Wide Web) and when one area of the network has a failure, the entire network is affected. This is exactly like the effects of a stroke. Living with a recovering brain is weird and something I navigate in every waking moment. As I edit this section, I consider myself very lucky in terms of my physical recovery, but the internal recovery (i.e. the mental, emotional and spiritual) is ongoing. Again, I count myself lucky. Thanks to the incredible support of my love, Claire, I have navigated the mental, emotional and spiritual roller coaster that has allowed me to play an active, albeit different, role in the world.

Experiencing brain damage (also known as a Traumatic Brain Injury) may sound like there is no hope, but that is far from the case. Hope comes in the form of the scientific term, Neuroplasticity, and one's perspective on life. Neuroplasticity, which is in all of us, is the fundamental ability of the brain to rewire itself and form new neurology. It is something that occurs in every one of us and it's happening all the time without our conscious awareness. Neuroplasticity is the scientific key to recovery and change. Perspective is very personal. That concerns one's outlook on life. It's profound across many dimensions and reaches into unproven territory that our logic-based science can yet prove or test, and when those subjects and ideas are beyond our mainstream sciences then our willingness to "go there" is often challenged. Perspective and one's outlook on life have a significant impact on one's life and in my experience, contain the most powerful form of hope.

Like many others who have experienced a near-fatal, life-changing event, the world never appears the same again. The level of change in that respect is different for everyone; it's a very personal thing. Nonetheless, one's worldview changes in that instant and thereafter.

When I consider my life pre-stroke and then post-stroke, there is a very different realisation. Pre-stroke, I used to reflect on myself as friendly, positive, open-minded, a lover of nature and enthusiastic about most of what life had to offer. Post-stroke, those attributes have not gone, but they have been augmented with a depth of understanding that influences how I approach the world and my relationship with myself, and therefore others. This understanding manifests in a way that I can only theme as "life is beautiful in all its forms and it is for living/experiencing."

Those words don't do this newfound understanding justice. They are very human, surface-level words. The depth in my heart for life and appreciation for everyone and everything is almost indescribable. I suppose it is a deeply felt love for literally everything in the world and beyond. I feel the love of a universal God energy in my heart and that then emanates in all that I am and all I can be and do. This is a God energy that is not tied to any religion or man-made set of rules. It is much more than anything man-made. I see the love and the beauty in everyone and everything. I have to admit that pre-stroke maybe I wasn't like that. I wonder to myself, did I judge others in the same way I used to judge myself? I hope not and I truly never meant any harm to others if I did. But today, post-stroke, all that has gone. I'm a different person. And that is a gift!

Everything has slowed down to a pace where I can truly appreciate the beauty and the perfection in the unfolding of the life experience. Life is so precious and I used to be guilty of always thinking of the future, and unable to fully appreciate the present moment.

Having a brain haemorrhage called a stop to that kind of future-only-based thinking in an instant. I was knocked off my feet as a 4cm area of blood burst into my cerebellum whilst hundreds of people around me carried on with their lives having fun at a rugby cider festival. No one knew (or could know) what was happening in my brain. I didn't know! It was about as untimely as you can get, although let's be honest, there's never a good time to have a brain haemorrhage is there? It could be described as indiscriminate and random or I might have manifested it into my physical reality, but whatever, it happened, it was most definitely "a thing".

But God's plan included the fact that I wasn't supposed to die on that life-changing day. If I was meant to die at 53 years of age, that would have been the moment. But I was gifted another chance at life.

As I first became aware of my situation in the early days of hospitalisation I started to imagine a book that told this story. A book that allowed me to chart this journey of recovery; this transformation and document the life lessons that I hope others can learn from too, not just survivors of stroke and brain injury, or immediate loved ones and family, but anyone who is willing to learn from such an event.

As mentioned previously, I refer to God (e.g. God's plan) as a simple reference to an infinite intelligence that is all around and in all of us; in all and everything in the entire universe (physical and spiritual). This is not something external, but rather something omnipresent; present everywhere, in everything, in everyone and at all times.   I am not religious, although I am baptised and confirmed Christian within the Church of England, where God is worshipped as a metaphorical 'he', as God The Father. But I have experienced a change in my life that has resulted in my rediscovery of my connection to my God-self within the context of an omnipresent life force. By God-self I refer to the love and light that is deep within every living thing in the physical and spiritual universe. As a result of this entire experience, I have come to a point of remembering that everyone and every living thing possesses that God-spark, that God-self, but I, like many, had lost that in my former (pre-stroke) years. My deepest wish is that you can perhaps rediscover your own God-spark as a result of reading this book and learning about my journey without having to go through such a potentially life-threatening event to do so.

The subtitle of the book states "...through the Law of Attraction." I do not blatantly promote any Law of Attraction rhetoric in this book, but anyone with even a limited understanding of the principles of that Universal Law will see it weaving throughout these pages as I chart and narrate my recovery journey. As I reflect on that journey it is apparent to me just how influential that Universal Law has been. It is now so obvious to me.

As you read, you will also, on occasion, see the word disease spelt dis-ease. This is deliberate and not a spelling error. The context will help explain why.

This is not a book that will project and preach at you. That is not my intention at all. It is simply an account of all of the events told in my style; sometimes sad, sometimes humorous, sometimes deep and weird, and sometimes stated in a very (almost blunt) matter-of-fact way. It is raw, honest and authentic in every way.

Finally, and most importantly, my sincere wish is that I hope you enjoy it and it touches something deep inside of you.

Preface - The Creation Of Me v3

Life can throw you a curve ball.

I think that's a fairly well-understood concept, right? You're merrily going along with life thinking things are generally okay; maybe there are some areas of life you think might need some work on or could be improved, but generally, things are okay... and then bang!! Everything "goes south"; tits up; down the toilet! You get my drift, the world gets turned upside down!

I lived a regular, normal life, although there were areas I would have liked to improve; probably plenty of areas to be frank, but I had my health, which I always stated was my number one priority, I had a great relationship after a painful divorce. My fiance, Claire and I, were blessed with success-fully blending 5 kids (4 of them under the age of 17) into our "blended" family unit. My health was a priority for me and I always thought that if I had my health then everything else could be worked on. As previously stated, I was in a wonderful relationship with Claire (and still am, thankfully),

I kept myself reasonably fit and strong, I would work out in the gym every day and eat healthily (on the whole), I didn't drink much alcohol, I didn't smoke...all the trademarks of a reasonably healthy lifestyle.

On September 11, 2021, that all changed in an instant. I had a brain haemorrhage which caused significant injury in the cerebellum area of my brain. The haemorrhage caused a 4cm area of blood to burst into my cerebellum (located at the back of the brain). Somehow, I survived, but it changed who I was from that day forward. I've reinvented myself from scratch. In the initial few weeks after the stroke I couldn't walk, I had lost my independence as a human being. I had become reliant upon others for all my needs. It was a hellishly frightening experience. Both the stroke itself, and the journey of recovery have been intense, but in taking the journey I have redefined who I am.

I rebooted my entire "operating system". I liken it to a software system upgrade. Since I was 14 years old I have been a bit of a techie, so the metaphor of system upgrade makes sense to me. I've always been a bit of a nerd. I remember I programmed a simple game when I was at school; I was aged 15. I left school at 16 with a bunch of O levels and CSEs and successfully secured an engineering apprenticeship. I was on day release to a technical college where amongst other traditional engineering subjects, I took microprocessing and robotics. I didn't particularly like the traditional engineering studies and work (except welding for some reason) but I excelled in the microprocessing class. I was the "go-to guy" for all my engineering college classmates when they needed help. Programming microchips and registers with logic gates and machine code made complete sense to me; it was easy... I told you I was a nerd! In the work setting at the company I worked for (as the apprentice), I moved into the computer department (known as ICT) and built a career in IT operations and end-user support and then later in the SaaS (software as a service) industry. I was a director in a software business that I co-founded with two others and then was a global Vice President in an international and well-respected software company leading a staff of over 140 across US and UK primary locations. This experience immersed me into the world of software, upgrades, updates, new releases and new versions for 30+ years in total.

So when my life was completely up-ended by the stroke, the notion of rebooting, or receiving a system upgrade initially helped me make some sort of sense of the situation. In this sense, I think of my childhood as version 1 of Me, and then my adult life pre-stroke as version 2 of Me. Post-stroke is now version 3 of Me (or Me v3).

In my mind, the reboot and system upgrade were an opportunity to fix old bugs and introduce new features (enhancements) in my being. In the software world, it is typical that with each new release or version of the software, there are accompanying release notes compiled by the programming team or developers. The release notes list and describe the fixed bugs and the new enhancements in that particular release or version of the software. I think that this is the case with me as well. That might sound odd to some people, but it works for me.

I've always liked to think of myself as being an optimist, although Claire might disagree. Overall, I've always had a positive outlook on life. I think it's fair to say that certain aspects of life would upset me and I would worry about the details or specific areas of concern, but overall, the outlook was positive. People would say that to me as well. For instance, perhaps after a presentation at an industry conference, people would come up to me and say, " I love your energy and positivity." I don't know, maybe it was a polite way of saying, "Your presentation was crap, but you were positive!" Haha, welcome to my sense of humour. But whatever the real reason, if things were going okay, I was generally a positive guy.

Let's get back to the reboot and system upgrade analogy.

Seeing this up-ended phase of my life as a reboot and system upgrade sat well with me (and still does) as I see that as a very optimistic thing. I mean wow, what an opportunity, right? Not everyone has the opportunity to hit the reboot button, get a shiny new upgrade and start over. The way I see this is that I've been gifted an opportunity to start over and create an entirely new version of myself. This is Me v3, so let's embrace it. Okay, so how it happened may not be ideal, but it is what it is, so let's embrace it!

As previously stated, I look at my childhood as Me v1, then my former adult life as Me v2, and now this is Me v3. Each version builds upon the past but it's an opportunity to drop some features, fix some bugs and introduce some amazing new enhancements.

In this sense, this gift of a reboot and system upgrade was/is an opportunity for a strong recovery and profound personal transformation. Recovery in the sense that certain core functions need to be restored and fixed, and profound personal transformation in the sense that exciting new features can be introduced and enjoyed. Wow, that is a cool thing, right?

Stroke can be very cruel, but for me and many others, the post-stroke version can be vastly better than the pre-stroke version. I have a huge belief in self-healing and a belief in the power of the mind. Mindset is everything when faced with a frightening situation such as recovery from a stroke (remember I spoke about perspective in the introduction).

I believe that my thinking can determine my future. Having a vision of a super healthy Me v3 helps me remain focused on the behaviours and actions that help to make that future a reality. It is very easy to succumb to feelings of fear and worry. Fear and anxiety are very powerful and they can take hold and derail me if I let them do so. But the choice is mine. I can choose to let fear and anxiety rule or I can choose the path of optimism, determination, grace and forgiveness.

I choose these four words carefully:

Optimism - I've already written about my optimistic outlook. This is a past feature from Me v1 and v2 that I'm choosing to take forward into Me v3.

Determination - This is another feature from Me v1 and V2 that I'm choosing to take forward into Me v3. I've always had a sense of determination, tenacity and adversity, to "get my head down" and do the work to get shit done. When I set my mind to something I (generally) do it. I've studied my human design and for those that are familiar with that belief system, I am a manifesting generator with a 1:3 profile. I've recognised that when my sacral (gut) gives me a full-blown YES then I put all my energy into any specific task. If my body (sacral/gut) says NO then forget it; it's not going to happen. I also have to temper this determination with my undefined heart which can lead me to prove my point on everything. This doesn't always serve me well and when I catch myself having to prove my point I have to control myself for that is my egoistic "not-self" taking over. However, overall, my determination has generally been a good thing for me so I'm choosing to take it forward with me into Me v3.

Grace - This is an entirely new feature of Me v3. Grace is something I've learned during this recovery. I've learned to have grace with myself and others. Grace in the sense that my awareness and understanding of myself and others have been honed and tuned. I've learned to have grace when I've not been able to accomplish tasks in the same way I used to. Grace comes in the form of kindness for myself and others. I've always liked to think I had a disposition for kindness and care to others so perhaps this is an enhancement rather than a whole new feature. With that said, the grace I now possess is more divine. It is almost impossible to describe this difference, but it is a heartfelt grace that emanates from the depths of my soul. This manifests in me in many ways; I'm a lot more authentic in my expression of love and compassion towards others; It's not that I didn't mean it before, but now it's from my very being; my soul; my purest heart.

Forgiveness - This is a new feature of Me v3. Had I been asked about my ability to forgive as Me v2, I would have said "Yes, of course", and I could cite numerous examples to back up that statement. But now I wonder if that forgiveness was like it is now; I'm not 100% sure. So what's different now? I think my judgement has disappeared which has led me to forgive myself for having previous judgments about all sorts of things, people and situations. So perhaps this sense of forgiveness is with myself and the world at large. I've learned acceptance and surrender; acceptance in that things are what they are, although I know I can change my circumstances if I choose to. So I accept people and external circumstances as they are without judgement and if I feel a sense of wrongdoing (which is an emotional reaction from my judgement) I witness it all with forgiveness of the thing and of myself for feeling that emotion. So Me v3 is learning to become the non-judgemental witness with forgiveness. You may notice that I said "learning to become". This is deliberate because this is an upgrade to Me v3 that is ongoing and not some one-off big-bang event.

As I conclude this section I am called to add two pieces of writing that I wrote during January 2022. They are reflective of the v3 of Me. I wrote one to be read in the morning and the other just before bedtime. I hope you enjoy these two pieces and if you also feel the calling, please use these yourself:

Today I choose...

Today is going to be a good day,
As I navigate this day, I choose to see,
Good from bad,
The light in the dark,
Clarity without uncertainty,
Abundance, not lack,
Gratitude rather than arrogance
The peace in the storm,
Strength not weakness,
Kindness, not hatred,
Understanding not resentment,
The beauty in all things,
Limitless potential,
Forgiveness without anger,
Ease rather than pain,
Love not bitterness,
Smiles in place of frowns
Truth not lies
Tenderness rather than aggression
Today, I will focus on these qualities of life
for they are all around if I choose to see them.

Simon Kent - 19 Jan 2022

Saying Goodnight...

This day is done.
It concludes another spin of the planet
through the Cosmos.
As I look back on the day I choose to focus
on the goodness of the day.
It is far too easy to let the not-so-good
dominate our thoughts.
But rather than focus on the
challenges and the upsets of the day,
Allow a moment to bask
in the light of goodness.
I choose to remember the moments that:
Brought me peace in my heart,
Made me laugh with joy,
Caused me to cry with tenderness,
Helped me understand a worldview
better than before,
Taught me compassion rather than intolerance,
Made me gasp in awe,
Allowed me to absorb the bliss,
Made me look with wonder,
Enabled me to experience the fun,
Caused me to Sing out loud,
Allowed me to love more.

Simon Kent - 19 Jan 2022

A Message To Other Survivors Of Stroke

This message was written for other members of a Facebook Group called Different Strokes which is linked to the UK charity of the same name. It's a Facebook community of 6800 members, mainly survivors of stroke of working age.

I wrote this on September 27, 2022, and if you are a stroke survivor reading this or having it read to you, this is for you too.

It's easy to get down after a stroke. It's normal to question "Why me?" and "What's going to happen now?"

Fear, worry and anxiety are all normal emotional reactions when surviving a massive brain trauma like a stroke.

We've all been there. Some of us are in that place right now. I hear you, I see you, I feel you.

But, never lose hope for the future. Will it be different? You can almost be certain that the answer to that is yes, but don't be afraid of that future. We are hurtling through space at over a million mph so change is and always has been uncertain, but inevitable, and all we have is now.

There is a beautiful Japanese word "Ikigai" which means "reasons for being".

When we are amid the raging storm, it's easy to lose sight of that "Ikigai", but one day it will return and it will light up your soul from the darkness and provide you with the fuel to carry on.

So live in the now moment, don't live in the past and know that one day the meaning behind all the madness will be revealed.

Sending love and light

Simon x

Buckle up and hold on tight, this is going to be the one heck of a ride!!

The Rugby
Festival

I

September 11, 2021

My family and I had decided to volunteer at the local rugby club. It was the 50th-anniversary festival for RWBRFC (Royal Wootton Bassett Rugby Football Club). William, my then 12-year-old son, played for the U12 team. To show our support for the club, we volunteered for BBQ duties in the late afternoon. Volunteering for various kitchen-type duties during training and matches was something I enjoyed so volunteering again for the festival was quite normal.

We arrived at 3:00 pm, the organiser of our volunteering team had told us to meet in the beer tent at 4:30 pm, so I thought I'd grab a quick pint beforehand thinking I didn't want much as I needed to be clear-headed for helping with the BBQ.

I had my one pint of Crazy Goat cider. It tasted quite strong and it was the strongest cider available at just over 6% alcohol.

I sipped my pint as I watched the senior team play against one of their rivals in the festival rugby fixture.

"Hmm, take it easy with this." I thought, so I nursed my single pint very deliberately, just gently sipping from the plastic glass.

At 4:30 p.m., we met in the cider tent for our volunteering duties. Claire and my daughter, Charlotte, went to the BBQ area, and I went to the bar area. I had never done any kind of bar duties before so I was a little nervous, but I thought, "What could go wrong, I'm only serving a few pints of cider or beer?" Also, Alfie, the husband of Lins (our U12's team manager), was on hand and helping behind the bar. So, although a little anxious, I believed I would learn the ropes pretty quickly.

Everything was going well. I was enjoying my inaugural bar duties and I was getting into the swing of it alongside my more seasoned volunteer bar staff.

One of my fellow servers, Cath, managed to squeeze a last 1/2 pint of Crazy Goat for us each, and not long after, Lins our organiser, fetched me a welcome pint of Cider from the bar of the main clubhouse.

I started drinking my Cider from the clubhouse before finishing the 1/2 pint of Crazy Goat... I don't recall ever finishing the Crazy Goat, or the Cider from the clubhouse, for that matter.

I should make it clear that I am not a big drinker. I'm not a big bloke (at a height of roughly 5' 6") and I don't like the feeling of being drunk at all, to be honest. Sure, loosening up a little was always a bit of fun, but not completely out of it. It's never been my thing.

So, picture the scene, I'm serving cider and beer in a beer tent at a local rugby festival. All is well with the world when suddenly out of nowhere...

... thwack! I felt a tremendous pain in the back right-hand side of my head. It felt like I'd been hit with a baseball or cricket bat. The pain was intense but I somehow remained standing. I squeezed the back of my head with my fingers in a vain attempt to quell the pain. I pushed my fingers into the back of my skull to stop the pain.

"What the hell was that?", I thought.

Simultaneously, I felt very "strange". My balance had gone completely. The pain was still there, but my overall sense was one of being completely disoriented.

I felt completely and instantly drunk!! So drunk that I could hardly stand.

Whoa, this was crazy!!

The effects of whatever it was took hold immediately, and everything got weirder and weirder very rapidly.

"This doesn't make sense," I thought. "I've had less than 2 pints so why do I feel so wrecked."

Everything changed so fast, this was the moment that my life would change forever.

2

Was I Really That Drunk?

I had never felt so wrecked in all my life. When I was younger I had experimented with various recreational drugs but the effect on my state of consciousness with this situation was something completely different. I was tripping out in a way I'd never experienced before, and I didn't like it; it was a very bad trip!

I quickly thought through all of the things I'd consumed that afternoon:

- 1 Pint of Crazy Goat Cider
- Then less than 1/2 Pint of Crazy Goat Cider (squeezed from the bag by Cath)
- Then less than 1 Pint of Cider from the clubhouse bar from Lins (probably about 1/2 Pint consumed)

- 1/2 Burger with Mustard (that Eva (my step-daughter) had given to me earlier)

"Was any of this poisoned?" I thought to myself.

"Had I been 'spiked' with something?" All manner of thoughts flew through my brain as I tried to make sense of what was happening to me.

"What? No, this was a family rugby anniversary festival at a local club, there wouldn't be any spiking going on here, surely not!"

Nothing made any sense. My brain was working through all the possibilities to try to find an answer to this madness.

I stood behind the bar, trying to adjust to the disorientation of my vision.

But still, nothing made sense, nothing at all and I couldn't see properly.

"What the fuck was happening?"

Everything appeared upside down. The world had shifted by 90 degrees. It felt like I was in some kind of washing machine!

I felt sick.

"No!" I thought to myself. "Not in the bar! Don't be sick in the bar. Imagine the embarrassment. Get out! Now!"

I looked over towards Claire and Charlotte and caught

Charlotte's eye. I tried to indicate that I felt really bad but did so by shaking my pint of (almost finished) Haze. Of course, poor Charlotte thought I was drunk. She laughed at me in a slightly embarrassed way, not able to make sense of why her Dad was acting so weird.

"No, I'm not drunk babe, there's something very wrong", I thought. But I couldn't communicate that at all. I didn't know what was wrong myself so I couldn't even begin to communicate it. I suspect that I probably couldn't have even found any words to articulate what was happening.

"I need help", my thoughts continued.

With a final thought of, "I need to get out of here", I started to make my way across the beer tent towards the BBQ area where Claire and Charlotte were working.

I stumbled through the beer tent and arrived at the table where Claire and Charlotte were cutting up bread rolls for burgers and hotdogs. I had made it to them! I was in one piece, without falling over, and without being sick...mission accomplished. But still, I felt awful.

They both looked at me with that look that said, "Really? What do you look like?"

"How much have you drunk?", Charlotte asked the question that they were both thinking.

I shrugged my shoulders and counted my fingers. It was all I could manage. I couldn't speak. I couldn't communicate with anyone about anything. I was in a big mess.

Claire left where she was working and came to support me. I felt an instant sense of comfort from her presence.

She would look after me and make everything ok.

I felt a bit like a little boy being tended to by his mother. I felt completely helpless and vulnerable. I wanted this to stop.

I was scared. I was really scared.

"Come on, let's get you back to the car", she said as she took me by my left arm, and we walked out of the beer tent.

We walked (or perhaps I should say we stumbled) together towards where we had parked our VW Transporter earlier that afternoon. I remember that I almost dragged my feet and had to lean on Claire a lot as we made our way towards our vehicle. I tried my best to not lean too heavily on Claire but had she not been by my side I wouldn't have known where I was going at all. I would have fallen flat on my face. I think she was doing pretty much all the walking and I was just blindly stumbling.

The next thing I recall is that Charlotte had joined us. We were by the van. Claire opened the tailgate so I could climb into the back. Our Transporter had one of those large up-and-over tailgate lids to enable easy access and standing room.

We had recently bought the VW as we had long-held dreams to convert it into a cool camper van. It was a Long Wheel Base (LWB) VW Shuttle Transporter. It was a mini-bus that can seat 9 people. We had removed the last row of seats and there was a makeshift bed in the back area with a couple of fairly long home-made cushions.

Claire laid out one of the long cushions on the floor and I crawled in. She left me with a bottle of water by my side. I was holding onto the bottle for dear life and I curdled up into the foetal position.

Claire and Charlotte, left me to "sober up". I was alone lying in the back of the van and I needed to pee!!

"Oh no, I can't just pee myself," I thought as I lay there alone, "I must get out of the van."

Luckily, Claire had left the tailgate open.

All I could do was shuffle myself down towards the open tail-gate. I tried to lean on my side but couldn't, I had no option but to shuffle in my foetal position.

"Whoa, what's happening to me?" I thought, followed quickly by "I can't even sit up to get out of the van. What the fuck!"

I managed to slide myself to the open tailgate, and then I slid onto the ground outside the van.

I couldn't see properly. I was forced to shut my eyes to block out the madness and stop myself from feeling sick.

I tried to open my eyes to get my bearings. I wanted to stand up and pee. I knelt forward, clenching my bladder muscles to stop me from peeing myself.

"Damn those ciders want to come out!", I thought to myself.

I tried to stand.

No way! I couldn't stand up. I figured that I would fall straight back down like a dead weight. There was no way on this earth that my legs would support me. I realised that I would have to crawl to pee somewhere.

I knelt up on one knee to get my bearings again. I looked over towards one of the rugby pitches near where we had parked.

I had a sense of how bad things were when I looked over towards the goalposts.

Rugby goalposts normally stand vertically parallel, like a big H shape in the ground. No, these were horizontally parallel! So the H had shifted by 90 degrees. Not only that, they were also slightly spinning circularly, but always parallel, nonetheless. I can only describe it as sheer hell! That may sound over dramatic, but when your entire reality is turned by 90 degrees and for no apparent reason, it is absolute hell on earth.

I rolled over backwards uncontrollably. I hit my head on the ground, hardened by the late-summer sun. Ouch! That hurt. I felt the thud reverberate around my head. I sensed a metallic taste or was it a smell? I couldn't ascertain whether it was a smell, a taste, or what; I didn't know what I could taste, smell, see, hear, touch; it was all utter madness.

With that, I heaved myself into a sitting position leaning against the rear of the van. Using my arms, I pushed myself into a seated position in the back of the open van and manoeuvred myself so that I could somehow relieve my aching bladder.

Finally, I could pee!

3

"Too Much Cider Then?"

I crawled back into the van. I must have passed out.

I became aware of the sound of Claire and Charlotte's voices back at the van. I couldn't make out what they were saying, although I do recall Claire asking if I was ok, and that she was going to take us all home.

Claire shut the tailgate and we set off across the grass. I was still lying in the back only dimly aware of the activities around me. Claire was collecting the rest of the kids from another area of the festival and then we were leaving the rugby club and on the road heading home.

I remember being able to see the trees going by as I lay in the back of the van. I was looking up trying to figure out where we were on our journey home.

We had arrived home and Claire turned off the engine.

Claire must have called ahead to her Dad, Roger.

"Aye up, too much cider then", Roger called out in his cheery Wiltshire manner.

I heard Claire speak to her Dad through the open window, "I'm going to need your help getting him into the house, please Dad."

I felt stupid! Probably a bit embarrassed if I'm honest, but I still couldn't explain what had happened.

They each took an arm and started to haul me out of the van.

"No, I'm going to be sick!", I said trying to be helpful.

Too late, I was sick in the back of the van.

"I'm sorry", I tried to say. I was embarrassed for being in such a state.

"It's ok", I heard Claire say in a caring, loving voice.

With Claire on one side and Roger on the other they managed to get me into the house, then into the downstairs toilet and then onto the sofa in the lounge.

Claire was an angel and stayed with me all night. She decided she needed to stay near me. I know she didn't get much sleep, that's for sure.

I slipped in and out of consciousness all night.

I would wake, need to be sick in a washing up bowl, need the toilet and then slip back into unconsciousness (or sleep, as we thought).

In the initial stages, Claire (and everyone else) thought it was a very bad case of being drunk, but I seemed to be getting worse rather than better. With alcohol, the effects of being drunk eventually fade away. But not with this. Not with me. I was getting worse if anything. I couldn't open my eyes, I was sick, my head was pounding and there was no way I could stand up.

At some point during the night, I told Claire about rolling and hitting my head on the ground at the back of the van. Her thoughts turned to a concussion or some other form of head injury. Her concerns were heightened.

Claire called the 111 service and then the Ambulance Service at around 3 a.m.

I drifted in and out of consciousness for the remainder of the night. The cycle would go sleep, wake up, retch to be sick, toilet, back to sleep, probably every 20-30 minutes, perhaps less, I'm not sure.

An ambulance arrived at the house at about 7:15 a.m. Yes, 4 hours and 15 minutes after being called!

The crew were quite dismissive of my condition and stated that they thought it was a severe case of vertigo.

I can only assume that either I did something or Claire said something that made them take me to the hospital, as the next thing I recall is being strapped to a type of wheelchair and being pushed out of the house and into the back of the ambulance.

Claire kissed me goodbye and the kids were also there, and then the ambulance doors shut, I don't remember anything else...

Hospitals

4

Darn! I'm High Up!

At this point, in the early part of this story, things become slightly fragmented and blurred. Somehow, I had survived an extreme form of brain injury and I had sustained damage to former healthy brain neurology and tissue.

Life had taken a huge change in direction.

I regained consciousness for a short while in the Great Western Hospital (GWH) in Swindon.

I remember opening my eyes and realising that I was in a hospital ward. I wasn't concerned. I felt a sense of peace because I was in the hospital.

I looked around the ward and realised I was in a corner bed. I could see the sky out of the far window on the opposite side of the room. I could sense that the ward was situated high above the ground floor. I could also see the countryside on the eastern side of Swindon. I could see where the sky met the rolling countryside hills. I knew the area I was looking at but couldn't remember the names of the villages in that area. I do recall that the landscape was horizontal and not vertical anymore so that was a blessing. Some sense of normality had returned, I was not vomiting any more and my headache had subsided.

Claire was with me. She said I was going to be transferred to Oxford.

I'd had an immediate CT brain scan when I was admitted to GWH which showed that I'd had a bleed on my brain.

My thoughts immediately turned to a distant memory and recollection from my childhood of a man in his thirties who lived in the same village as my family and I. One night an ambulance had taken him away. Later that same day, we heard that the man had a brain haemorrhage during the night. He never returned. Sadly, he died. I remember thinking, "People die from a brain haemorrhage."

I remembered this memory when I was told about my haemorrhage. This was not a good situation, but somehow I was alive.

Claire went on to say that someone called Amy had told her that GWH had sent CT images to John Radcliff University Hospital in Oxford and that the specialist team in Oxford had said that they wanted me there in their care at Oxford.

Bleed on the brain? I couldn't comprehend what I was being told. I was at the point of beyond caring. The sun was shining as I looked out of the window. I was in a blissful state of peace.

The former feelings of hell had stopped. I didn't feel sick anymore. The horizon was the horizon again. In that moment I was ready to die for all I cared. I was truly in the hands of God; I surrendered to the peace.

I passed out again.

I later found out that Amy was an amazing nurse in GWH who had seen me and helped with my immediate care as soon as I arrived at the hospital. She was also there to give loads of help and support to Claire. As it had been over 13 hours since the brain haemorrhage had occurred, there was no medical treatment, no surgery, no special medication, nothing. Throughout the entire time, I had been in the hands of God and I had no choice whatsoever but to surrender completely. I had CT scans and various other procedures to assess my condition and it could have gone either way at that point, live or die. Somehow, I lived.

I awoke to the sense of being wheeled in a bed through the corridors of the hospital and then into the back of an ambulance.

I recall an ambulance paramedic crew of a man and a woman, probably in their thirties. The woman stayed with me in the back of the ambulance while the man went to drive. They were taking me to Oxford.

I could just make out that we were joining the M4 Motorway at J15, we were moving at high speed. I tried to listen for the sound of the siren but couldn't hear it at all. I concluded that either the siren was off or that the back of the ambulance was soundproof so as not to scare travelling patients even more than they already were. It's weird what thoughts went through my head on that journey to Oxford.

I wasn't scared. I felt safe. I had no idea what was going on I suppose.

I tried to figure out where I was on the journey to Oxford, but could only see treetops flashing by quickly. I quickly gave up and I passed out again.

5

Oxford University Hospitals - John Radcliff

I arrived at Oxford without really any comprehension of what was happening, where I was going or what state I was in.

I recall that Claire visited me in the evening (Sunday, September 12, 2021) but I have only a vague recollection of that first day and evening in Oxford.

On Tuesday, September 14 I was aware of being wheeled to an operating theatre to have a procedure called a Brain Angiogram. It's a procedure that helps Neurologists determine the condition of blood vessels and, in my case specifically, the blood vessels in the cerebellum area of my brain.

The procedure is such that a catheter is inserted into the

Femoral Artery and dye is released into the bloodstream once the catheter has reached the area of concern. In my case, this was in my brain. The die is then used to help determine the condition of blood vessels via a scan.

I recall a surgeon speaking to me as I was lying in the operating theatre. There were a lot of people around dressed in blue gowns, some in green gowns and others with white tops and blue trousers.

The surgeon said something like, "So Simon, we're just going to send a small device into you so that we can look around and see what's going on." He then added, "You will be awake but don't be concerned as we will numb the area in your groin where we go in. You might feel a small sensation as we travel up from your groin through your body, and you might have a slight metallic taste, but this is all very normal."

Under normal circumstances, I think I would have freaked out and said, "WTF! You want to insert a catheter into my body at my groin and then push it through my body and up into my brain…and I'm going to be awake!! Are you fucking kidding me? No way!"

But I was in no state to resist. Quite the opposite.

I had a huge wave of acceptance and surrender wash over me. That entire team of medical professionals could have done anything to me and I wouldn't have cared in that moment. They were brilliant and I felt cared for and in very safe hands.

God was working miracles through this incredible team of medical professionals and all I could do was surrender.

As the procedure was underway, I didn't feel a thing. I suppose I must have felt the local anaesthetic being injected into my groin area, but in all honesty, I can't even remember that.

The only recollection I have of the procedure is a very strange sensation in my throat as the catheter was fed further into my body towards my brain. It's so weird when I type this now, but it's also rather like one of those wow moments in my life that I don't ever wish to repeat, still, it was one hell of a crazy experience!

With the procedure finished, I was wheeled back to my private room in a hospital ward in an unfamiliar place in a city far away from home, but at that time I didn't care, I was being looked after. It was like complete and utter surrender on my part.

The remainder of my time in John Radcliff Hospital was punctuated by Claire visiting me, and with food (breakfast, lunch, dinner).

Most of my time spent there is a blur. The dates were September 12 - 19, 2021. Our very good friends, Gemma and Kevin, gave Claire car lifts between our home and John Radcliff Hospital in Oxford for that entire week, they were amazing and I am so grateful for their generosity of time and energy (and fuel).

Throughout my stay in Oxford, I recall expecting that Claire would visit although I had no sense of time passing except by the punctuation of meals.

I remember the first occasion when a kind person asked me what meals I would like to order. I didn't have a clue! They proceeded to read out to me various options. Again, I didn't have any idea or concept of what was being discussed. I just grunted something that must have resembled a "Yes, please" and so my meal order was complete, I guess I'd find out later what would arrive.

I was due to start a large consultancy contract with a global client on September 13, 2021, but clearly, all those plans were shelved and my contract was eventually given to someone else to fulfil. The nature of being your own boss is that there are great risks.

Looking back now, I wish I had insured myself for such a life-changing event, but of course, hindsight is such an exact science. Before this period in September 2021, any thoughts of stroke never even entered my head, so I didn't have any critical illness insurance at all.

6

"I'm Surprised You Didn't Get Up!"

I recall one morning one of the nurses talking to me, she said something like, "Oh, I'm surprised you didn't get yourself to the bathroom last night."

That was it. I heard that innocent phrase and idle chat as an instruction. She didn't mean that I should get up to my bathroom at night. She was only joking. But my brain took it as a direct instruction! I took it as "I must get up and take myself to the bathroom during the night. That is what they expect of me. It's part of my recovery."

When I consider that I was in a private room in a ward within one of the main neuroscience centres of the UK which is all part of the prestigious University of Oxford Hospital, and it was only a couple of days since I had survived an almost fatal brain haemorrhage, I suppose the chances of a leading UK medical professional suggesting to me that I should get myself up to the toilet at night alone is rather ridiculous. Nonetheless, my injured and very confused brain took it as an instruction.

The nurse was a lovely, caring person and exceptionally brilliant at her job. Had she realised that my injured brain would take the joke as an instruction, then I know she wouldn't have said it, but she couldn't possibly know how my brain would react. I would like to emphasise that she is an outstanding professional and I take full responsibility for my brain and the events that later ensued.

The following night, I suppose it might have been the night of Wednesday, September 15, 2021, I set a plan to go to the bathroom to empty my bladder in the toilet, rather than use the supplied cardboard pee bottles.

I was in a private side ward with my own bathroom.

I dropped off to sleep as usual. I wasn't yet bothered about TV, iPhone, Books or any other form of entertainment; I was just in a state where I drifted in and out of consciousness; Claire would visit, I would have a meal and then back to sleep again. It was only the fact that the lights were switched off and the blinds at the window were shut that I had any awareness at all that it was nighttime.

At some point in the night, I awoke and I remembered my

plan for the bathroom. Yes, I needed to get to the bathroom, and I had been given my instructions. So like a good soldier, I had to comply; it was my duty; I must do this.

I was dressed in just a hospital gown which I was wearing backwards; I didn't realise it was backwards at the time, I just thought that's how they were. In the following weeks, I would later discover that this is not the case. Anyway, on this particular night, I was wearing one backwards so my arms were inserted and it covered my front but none of the buttons were done up at the back, which I didn't comprehend at the time.

I looked at my target; the bathroom door on the far side of my private ward. I studied my current location; I was in a bed wearing a gown. I knew I couldn't walk; it would be crazy to even try as I would fall into medical equipment and cause chaos.

My bed was surrounded by all sorts of medical kit but I was not attached to any of it. I was free but unable to walk because of my brain injury.

Ok, I thought, the plan is to crawl on my hands and knees; so I did precisely that.

I set off on my quest for the bathroom; I was determined to do it. I suppose it was the equivalent of setting off to climb Everest or something equally monumental and crazy. Somehow, I clambered out of the bed and onto the floor. Silently, without causing any noise or drawing any attention from the on-duty night shift nurses, I started to crawl across the floor on my hands and knees, but there was a problem.

The gown started to fall forward. As I wasn't aware of the buttons being at the back and the fact that they were not fastened, this had not been in the plan! My knees caught on the loose material gathering beneath me; I was going to fall onto my face if I wasn't careful. I tried to continue by gathering up the loose material in a way that would still allow me to crawl, but quite frankly it was not going to work.

I decided to take the gown off completely.

So there I was crawling across the floor of my (luckily) private room. I was completely naked but determined to reach my target of the bathroom toilet. I can imagine the sight! Not pretty at all! Of course, by this time I needed to pee as well but I managed to block any sensation of needing to pee by focusing on the target; this was a mighty quest that I had to accomplish, naked or not, it didn't matter to me either way!

I got to the bathroom door. I reached up and opened the door and was able to pull on the bathroom light cord. All good so far, I had arrived at the destination and it was now illuminated. Brilliant!

I then realised that the toilet was higher than I was as I was still crawling on the floor. Mmm, ok, what now? I thought to myself. I could sit on the toilet I suppose, that would work. I knew full well that standing was going to be impossible, but sitting was a possibility I suppose. My brain was trying to think on the fly and come up with solutions to my immediate problems.

I crawled towards the toilet, and using the toilet as leverage, I started to pull myself onto the toilet. I didn't have the strength to pull myself up, and massive dizziness kicked in to make the entire bathroom and toilet spin. I fell backwards.

Luckily, I hadn't pulled myself very far at all as I had no strength, so I didn't fall far. Nevertheless, I still fell and rolled backwards.

Thump! I hit the back of my head on a solid concrete and brick wall near the opening of the bathroom door.

Ouch!

"Brilliant!" I thought to myself sarcastically.

"Well done Si, that didn't work very well did it?" was my next immediate thought. I continued the mental conversation in my head, "If you're not careful, you're going to injure yourself even more, you idiot, it's time to head back to bed. Abort the mission you fool; save yourself!"

Still naked, I crawled back across the floor to my bed. I collected my crumpled gown on the way.

On arrival at my bed, I looked up at my new target (the bed) from the height of the floor. "How the heck am I going to get back on there?" I thought to myself.

Somehow, I managed to crawl back onto the bed, with my gown, and I was hugely relieved to be back in safe territory; I had made it back into my bed in one piece and I could use the cardboard pee bottle to relieve myself; what an adventure, and no one knew, and I didn't need rescuing.

The next morning the same nursing professional came in to check on me at the start of her day shift. I told her about my mission to get to the bathroom. I remember being very proud of myself as I recalled all the details to her. She explained that she didn't mean for me to undertake such a task, especially alone at night but I was so proud of myself and couldn't wait to tell her the story of my adventure.

Later that day when Claire came to see me, the nurse told Claire all about my nighttime antics. Claire said to me that she had told the nurse, "Oh that sounds about right. That sounds like the sort of thing Simon would do!" I remember that even though both the nurse and Claire were questioning my sanity, the feeling of accomplishment far outweighed any feelings of embarrassment and regret. To me, even though the mission had to be aborted and I had to pee in a cardboard pee bottle, it was still a huge success. I can't to this day explain why. I suppose it was a significant early milestone and it was a reflection of my determination to overcome anything, despite the adversity.

7

God is a guy called Jacob

Later that night, the nurse had left to go home and a new head nurse, Jacob, was in charge of the night shift.

I realised that I was appreciative of being in a private ward alone. The noise of a public ward was diminished significantly when the door was shut, and this was especially beneficial at night time. If I needed anything all I had to do was press my buzzer which I could reach from the bed, and then someone would come to help. It was an ideal set-up. I was alone, the door would get shut and the outside noise of the ward would be shut out, and then someone would come in if I needed help. I was so grateful for that setup.

A nurse came in to give me some medicine and she walked out without closing the door. I pressed the buzzer and she returned about 5 minutes later. I asked if she could close the door, please.

"I'm afraid I can't, sorry", she replied.

"What?, No!!", I thought to myself.

I enquired why it was not possible and stressed how important it was for me. I knew that my body needed to heal and I instinctively knew that I wanted plenty of sleep for that healing to take place. I also knew that the chances of a good night's sleep were vastly reduced with the door left open. The sound of the main ward outside with its constant noise of buzzers, bleeps and alarms was not going to help with sleep at all. I felt a sense of panic within my body.

"Oh no, why not? Please can you shut it, I need the sleep.", I was almost pleading and begging.

'I'm sorry", she said, and added, "The head nurse has said that the door must be left open tonight because you got out of bed last night."

"Oh no!", I thought, "I only got up because the other nurse told me to!", at least that's what my injured brain was telling me. My mind was racing and I was getting frustrated with the situation.

I realised that it was pointless trying to argue my case with the nurse, so I asked, "Who is the head nurse please?"

"Jacob", she replied.

"Ok, great, could I speak with Jacob please?", I asked.

In that moment and the next hour, whilst waiting for Jacob to come and see me, I realised that nothing else in my world mattered. In that moment God was this guy called Jacob.

Jacob became the central linchpin and the deciding factor of whether I was going to have my much-needed healing rest that night, or not.

It's strange how the mind reacts in these types of situations. In my mind, my entire well-being rested with Jacob. He was EVERYTHING in my world at that specific moment; he was God and the centre of my universe at that hour. His decision would determine my fate. Nothing else mattered but Jacob.

Jacob walked into my room. He had a pleasant smiling face.

"Hello Simon", he said.

I greeted him and we discussed the situation. He explained that because I had got out of my bed the previous night they must keep the door to my room open. "For my safety", was the phrase he used.

I understood the argument but I explained how I desperately needed my sleep and that I would not be repeating the same stunt; after all, it wasn't successful anyway and I had learned my lesson.

I must have said something right, because he agreed with me and agreed to allow the door to be closed.

YES!!

It was a sweet victory and I slept so well; fully relaxed with immense gratitude for Jacob and my quiet private room with the door shut.

The remainder of my time in Oxford passed without any more excitement or incidents. I recall that all the doctors, nursing, cleaning and volunteer staff were lovely and kind. I tried to get to know each person, what was their name and anything about them. I would test myself to see if I could recall any of the information and for the time whilst I was there, I think I was pretty successful; alas, today, most of those lovely people are now a distant memory, but my gratitude for the love and care that they gave me is boundless.

My recovery in Oxford concluded on September 19. I was to be sent back to Swindon. I was to be repatriated, as they called it.

I find it interesting that even in those very early days of re-covery, I had started to envision that this story would be told. I imagined a book and a film, so who knows where this might go. In my mind at the time, I felt that the situation that I had found myself in and the circumstances of the rugby festival must be told. If for no other reason than to raise awareness with others that someone who is having a brain haemorrhage and a stroke will look very weird. In my case, I looked drunk, but each situation is unique because everyone is unique; their brains are unique and when a stroke occurs the circumstances are unique. Be aware!

Transformation Key: Transformation takes determination. Find grace for yourself as you face hardships. Forgive yourself and others when you feel in a low vibrational energy (mood). You're lucky to be alive. Love yourself. You are worthy.

8

⚜

Swindon - Great Western Hospital (Swindon GWH)

I remember the journey back to Swindon from Oxford, although I had no recollection of particular landmarks on a road I was very familiar with. I was wheeled into the back of a community ambulance so there were no blue lights or sirens on this occasion, thank goodness.

"I'm back in the same ward I was in last week", was my immediate thought as I was wheeled into a ward in GWH (Great Western Hospital), Swindon.

It felt great to be back on home ground. I think it made a huge difference to Claire as well as she was able to visit me much easier. She was no longer reliant upon the generosity and kindness of Gemma and Kevin; for transporting her to and from Oxford.

I was still pretty much out of it, to be honest. I remember Claire saying something about it being easier to visit which made sense at the time, but I was so ill, I didn't register or feel the benefit personally, but I was pleased for Claire as she seemed a bit more relieved.

Claire was amazing; she always visited; it became quite a highlight of my day and routine.

I spent just one week in GWH whilst I undertook initial physiotherapy and in that time more tests were conducted on me to determine the overall cause of the brain haemorrhage. As no root cause was found, it was concluded that the likely cause was hypertension (high blood pressure).

In my time at GWH, I predominantly slept, but I also started to see signs of progress as each day passed. It was whilst at GWH that I started to post about my recovery on social media

There were multiple reasons for posting:

I wanted to tell my story and warn people about the dangers of stress, high blood pressure and hypertension.

I also wanted to record my progress as I knew that one day I'd write this story and my memory would not remember the detail like it was in the moment. So in that way, it provided me with a social diary and journal which in turn, provided me with a facility to look back and recall the details.

At the time, I had no idea of the positive impact my posts would have and how people would react. I wasn't seeking any reaction at all, except maybe to warn people of stress and high blood pressure.

It transpired that people were very supportive and appreciated my honesty, transparency and authentic style. My posts have always been from the heart. I didn't have the energy to plan or stage-manage my posts; they just spilt out in the moment; and continue to do so to this day.

So with that said, the next section of this story is guided by those social media posts that journaled my recovery. As I have reproduced the posts in this book, I've also provided an additional narrative that describes the backstory to the specific post or elaborates upon the message, along with an associated Transformation Key which I hope you enjoy.

The Transformation Key is a simple line or two of wisdom that encapsulates the essence of the journal entry and the additional narrative.

Writing this section of the book has been an interesting and very cathartic exercise and has in itself offered yet deeper levels of personal emotional healing. As the Transformation Keys have been written, I have captured all of them in another series of books of that same name. The idea is that transformation is universal and not only limited to stroke survivors.

Transformation Key: Chart your progress; You will be amazed at your transformation.

9

23 September 2021: F..K That Hurts!

> *Stomach cramps in a hospital bed be like... "F..K THAT HURTS!!"*

I recall lying in my hospital bed and I had to move; I needed to sit up slightly. I engaged my stomach muscles and the worst cramp hit my stomach. It was awful. All I could do was grip my stomach with my hands and fingers in a useless attempt to stem the cramps. I was digging my fingers into my stomach muscles to find some much-needed relief from the intense pain. Nothing worked.

Eventually, I breathed my way through it.

The cramp was bad; I had experienced it before, but what

made it worse was that I couldn't move. I was bedridden and unable to move at all. Whilst the cramp prevented any kind of movement anyway, the fact that I couldn't move at all seemed to make the situation a whole lot worse. It wasn't any fun at all!

Transformation Key: The power of breath will amaze you.

10

❧

24 September 2021: A New Day And New Goals

A new day and new goals....

As I recover in hospital from this stroke that nearly took my life, I give grace and thanks to God for being gifted a second chance.

Each day brings forth a new set of challenges that I must accomplish with ease in order to return where I want to be most, home with my family and in the loving arms of my love Claire

I have many goals for the future but today the focus is:

Independently get myself to the toilet

Independently wash

Write this post

Write a chapter in my forthcoming book

> *Kill it in today's physiotherapy session*
> *Wishing everyone a great day*

This post from early in my recovery captures several important aspects.

I intuitively knew that I was lucky to be alive. As I was lying in my hospital bed I had no idea of the statistics associated with stroke but I realised that there was a significant chance of immediate death from a brain haemorrhage. I was so very lucky to be alive.

I've always been a spiritual person but I suppose if I'm honest with myself, I hadn't spoken about my spirituality or my faith to very many people at all. I had spoken openly to Claire and my mother, but no one else. I think this post was probably the first time I had spoken openly and publicly about God. I wasn't trying to make a point but it just felt right; it felt natural to do so. I was alive and I naturally felt the presence of God (or a higher life force and divine intelligence) in that moment.

There's also an aspect in that post that reflects my determination again.

I am a very goal-oriented person; I like to achieve things; I've always been that way I suppose. So it felt normal to me to start setting myself small goals to accomplish.

In that early stage of my recovery, regaining my independence was an important priority for me. My rationale went something like this:

Claire is my fiance; she's my lover; she's not my carer. I didn't want her to help me go to the toilet or bathe; she didn't sign up for that. I know people in love will do all manner of tasks for their loved ones and that is a beautiful thing but I didn't want that for Claire. I don't think anyone wants to become reliant upon anyone else for their personal hygiene needs; I think the human condition of self-reliance is very strong But of course, many others are not as fortunate as I was. I knew that I could win this internal battle with myself. I was not going to lose. Claire was not going to be my carer; she was my fiance, and that was that! I realised early in my recovery that achieving goals might take me some time and I accepted that, but determination was a hallmark of my character that seemed to show itself when I needed it, and this was one of those moments.

Equally, alongside determination, I'd say that other overriding aspects of my recovery have been, and still are, surrender and acceptance. Many words come to mind: resilience, fortitude, determination, strength, surrender, acceptance, forgiveness and grace, but the most powerful word of all is love.

Self-love (or self-care) has played a very important part in my recovery. I mean this primarily in the mental and emotional sense, and I truly believe that my spirituality and faith in a higher life force and divine intelligence (God is an okay word if you want) have contributed greatly to my discovery of inner peace throughout my recovery from this life-changing stroke.

The early signs of this book were sprouting on September 24, 2021. Today it is February 18, 2022. The book is not finished but it's underway. I am determined to finish it and tell this story. It is now October 18, 2022, as I review and edit the initial written words.

Transformation Key: You're alive; Learn to surrender and accept what is; You can find peace where you are right now; You are on a journey

11

24 September 2021: A Second Chance

God has given me a second chance:
The sun is brighter
The grass and flowers smell sweeter
The air is fresher
Conversations are richer
Life has a brilliance that is almost palpable
God, I promise I'll do my part in reaching the targets that shows
I am worthy of this second chance
Just name the goal, I'll do the work...
I posted earlier today listing my goals for today. I have smashed them all
it feels F***ing amazing
A Dr said yesterday that my target BP is 130/80, a nurse just

came to monitor it and it read 138/82 boom almost there, I'll take that.

2 weeks ago it was crazy high well over 200

Also today, the physio therapy team had me walking up/down the ward corridor - I am having to relearn mobility before I can leave for home.

This means that they take off the very weird electro stimulus devices on my legs (that prevent DVTs) - these are essential but definitely don't help towards a peaceful nights sleep

which is the best medicine of all.

More updates to come tomorrow

Onwards and upwards

Stay tuned .....

Once again, God is featured in my posts from the hospital. I couldn't smell the grass, flowers or fresh air while I was in the hospital but they were all those things in my mind; my third eye; my imagination was creating a new, richer world and I was ready to do the work to bring it all into my reality.

Once it was established that hypertension caused the brain haemorrhage then I was prepared to do whatever it took to lower and stabilise my blood pressure. Blood pressure is a regular feature of my life now (over a year later) and I suspect that I will monitor it regularly for the rest of my life.

I recall having to wear various types of electronic stimulus devices on my lower legs whilst I was lying in bed not moving.

The doctors on the ward were concerned that I might develop a Deep Vein Thrombosis (DVT). I can't remember the name of the first device but I do recall that eventually, I progressed onto things called Gekos. I guess they performed their job well but it was almost impossible to get a good night's sleep whilst wearing the Gekos. Every 10 seconds or so, I would receive an electric pulse (or shock) in my lower legs which would result in a severe twitch or spasm in both feet and lower legs. I recall Claire coming to visit and seeing my legs and feet twitching uncontrollably. "What's going on with your legs? Are you okay?", she remarked. "It's these weirdo Gego things", I replied and proceeded to explain their function to Claire.

Transformation Key: Your imagination is so powerful; Put it to work and imagine the beautiful future that you can create; This current reality will pass.

12

25 September 2021: Anton

Amazing conversation with Anton from Physio Therapy this morning.

When he first met me last Wednesday, I could only walk with the help of two people, today I'm walking, washing etc independently. 3 days!

I get impatient with myself as my goals are far greater than Independent washing etc but like all goals I have to learn the baby steps first.

I cannot wait for where this journey takes Claire Chapman and I

Nothing happens to us, it always happens for us!

Onwards and upwards

Be grateful for everything in your life and celebrate every

> *small step*
> *Ps. I also managed to get into my own PJs and GnR t-shirt today (rock n roll)*

The physiotherapy team in the GWH at Swindon were remarkable. They are so patient and kind with people like me who were having to re-learn how to walk, move around and establish independence.

Nothing can prepare you for the madness that ensues after a stroke. Everyday tasks like walking to the toilet become major milestones. It seems almost ridiculous really but it's true, with patience the tasks can become normal again and the muscle memory does return as the brain heals itself.

There's something that Anton (Lead Physio Therapist) said to me whilst I was relearning to walk. He said, "Walking is like controlled falling". I think that is brilliant advice and it will stick with me forever; I will never forget that. That phrase helped me tremendously. As I took my first tentative steps I had that phrase running through my head. I'm not quite sure exactly how it helped, but it helped.

In my early days of physiotherapy, it was really hard. All I wanted to do was rest; I didn't want to do the work but something made me do it (besides the physiotherapists being insistent). My self-determination also helped. Despite the pull to stay in bed and the excuses running through my head; "too tired" was always an excuse that worked and caused people to leave me alone. But I thought to myself, "That's ridiculous, who am I kidding here? They are trying to help me. Now just get on with it and stop making excuses!"

I would have these internal mental battles quite a lot. It's so tempting to give up, but that doesn't result in anything. I figured, "Well if I try and fail at least I've tried." So I did just that, I tried. And yes, it made me tired. No, it made me exhausted actually. I would sleep for hours afterwards. It took every ounce of energy out of me. I didn't realise it at the time but this was my first introduction to brain fatigue.

Through my determination and the care and guidance of the physio team, I made great progress. Within 3 days of starting physio, I was walking and washing independently; it was working!! It was 2 weeks after my stroke and I could now walk to the bathroom and wash independently. For 1 week I was only able to crawl to the bathroom and then not use the toilet at all (remember the story from Oxford?) This was recovery starting to take shape. When help is offered, take it.

Transformation Key: FAIL means First Act In Learning; It's great to fail, it means you are learning.

13

25 September 2021: 2 Weeks Ago

This time 2 weeks ago I suffered an almost life-ending stroke. Thanks to the intuitive actions of Claire Chapman and the incredible NHS, the outcome is that I'm still here and preparing to go again at this magic called life.

I tell this tale as one of caution and awareness so that others might also benefit from swift action.

It started at the local community's 50th anniversary rugby festival (go # RWBFC). There was cider and ale flowing but I had volunteered myself and Claire for BBQ and bar duty so I deliberately restricted my cider intake to just one pint of Crazy

Goat cider.... I had no intention of getting pissed! In fact, I wanted to avoid that.

I had consumed my pint and by 4:30 pm we met to take our places in the bbq/bar.

By 6:30 pm it was game over. You would be forgiven thinking that I had continued to consume pint after pint of crazy goat, but no!! I had squeezed in another pint but not enough to give the effects I was experiencing- I was absolutely smashed - I couldn't see straight, I couldn't stand and it felt like I'd been hit around the back of the head with a cricket bat.

Holy shit what the hell was in this crazy goat had I been poisoned?

What the hell was happening to me? Nothing was making any sense whatsoever!!! I was scared!

I went to Claire, I needed help, She and Charlotte (my middle daughter) thought I was drunk so they thought that I should go to where we had parked the car earlier to sober up. Fair enough I thought..sounds like a plan.

I rolled around the ground, staggering and completely out of control - jeez this was embarrassing - way too much to drink!

Hours later I'm home and the so say "embarrassment antics continue", I've been sick my coordination is completely gone!

Claire and her Dad are doing their best to help me. By 3 am ish Claire's getting really concerned none of this was making any sense. She called an ambulance.

After a long night of sickness, sweating and severe headache, the ambulance arrived at 7:15 am on Sunday (over 12 hours since I first fell ill in the cider tent)

Claire was beside herself by this point, she knew something bad was going on but nothing made sense!!!! At this point, I was totally out of it....I was dying!

Only after arriving at Swindon A&E and having an MRI scan did anyone know that the situation was so serious ... the NHS KICKED INTO ACTION - this was a P1 emergency!

I was blue-lighted to Oxford and then spent a week with their neurological specialist care. Wow, I even remember the feeling of having keyhole imaging equipment enter my main artery and into my brain from my groin. That is proper crazy and all I could do was surrender to the situation- I was f...ked so I had no choice !!!! So, what's the point in this post? I guess there's so much to learn from this tale, I hope it serves that purpose - education perhaps. But the other aspect is one of judgement. To everyone else, I was literally blind drunk but what was

> *really happening was far far more severe.   So if you see someone in a mess maybe they're in desperate need so call an ambulance if you're in doubt. Listen to your intuition, it might save someone's life !!*

This post was an awareness and warning I suppose. I wanted to let people know how easy it is to misjudge someone who might be in desperate need of help. I looked like I was smashed drunk but I wasn't. Even the circumstance of a beer/cider festival at a rugby club would make people assume that I was just drunk but I wasn't, I was dying and about to experience brain damage and severe illness as I had never experienced before in my life; this was a life-changing event; I wasn't drunk. It would have been far easier if it had been a case of being drunk, but no, it was not that at all.

The message to anyone from this post is please don't judge what you think you see. We tend to judge and assume the worst and yet we have no conclusive evidence to support that judgement. We think we know. We think we've seen something. We think we've heard something. But have we? Really?

If someone had seen me in my 'state' they would have (understandably) assumed I was drunk. I was having a brain haemorrhage.

I don't hold any blame for anyone assuming incorrectly; being honest with myself I think I would have thought that too. But the lesson for anyone is never to judge what you think you witness.

I remember jumping to the conclusion that I had somehow been spiked or poisoned, because I had never experienced anything like it before, and neither had anyone else. The only experience like that, that I had had before was being drunk (not very often I might add) and add into that the association of a beer and cider festival at the local rugby club and hey presto, we have a classic scenario of pre-conceived ideas (i.e. judgement). We are all guilty of judging others, judging a situation, judging ourselves, and most of the time, we don't even realise we're doing it.

Luckily for me, the misjudgement wasn't fatal. But if it had been fatal, then no one would have been to blame or responsible. It was a collection of circumstances that all added up to be a misunderstanding, but clearly, God had other plans for me that day.

Transformation Key: Drop all judgment; Don't judge others and most of all, don't judge yourself

14

26 September 2021: Every Morning...

Every morning I have to walk up and down the ward.
The Physio Therapy team are brilliant
- they set the pace for rehabilitation - I love to be pushed - if I'm going to get on at home then I must be proficient with the basics. It's exhausting- the background work that the brain is doing is suddenly thrust into the foreground - arm swings, feet distance apart, focus on a point ahead, relaxing the shoulders, pace, you name it, it's got to be thought about and the brain has to figure it out... and at the same time hold a conversation.
We do this in our daily lives without any consideration or effort. As human beings we are amazing. It's ironic that it takes something so severe to realise how incredible we are.
Remind yourself today how incredible you really are !!!

As I underwent a physiotherapy routine imposed by the amazing team at GWH, it reminded me of just how amazing we are as human beings and we often don't release it; we forget just how brilliant we are.

Anton, who led the physio rehabilitation, was brilliant. He set the pace and pushed me when he knew I could do it.

He reminded me about the basics of walking that we just take for granted. He reminded me to fix my gaze on a point in front of me; I would use the clock on the ward wall or a sign in the corridor if I walked outside of my immediate ward area. I would have to deliberately swing my arm(s) and ensure my feet were not too far apart. I tended to walk like a robot to start with.

Before I met Anton, I had found a walking frame near my bed, so I used that as I started to navigate across the ward from my bed to the bathroom. When Anton first met me he said "Right, we'll take that frame away." I remember the feeling of frustration I felt, but he went on the explain that he didn't want me to become dependent on a frame. I understood his rationale and I didn't want that dependency either; he was right; I didn't need that; furthermore, I didn't want it.

As Anton and the physio team worked with me, I quickly made progress as I was determined to get the all-clear to go home. As I did the physiotherapy and retrained my brain to learn to walk again, I found it exhausting. Once I had finished I would sleep for hours.

The work that the brain is doing is nothing short of a miracle. It's working so hard to coordinate and send all the nerve signals to the right muscles and tendons. Balance, coordination, collision avoidance, risk assessment, arm swinging, focus on direction, target determination, feet correct distance apart, leg movement... the list goes on and on, and the brain is working on it all so quickly that it feels natural and we don't observe the sequencing, it all feels simultaneous and naturally coordinated and orchestrated. We forget how clever we are!! If you're having a bad day just remind yourself how amazing you are, and don't forget it!

Transformation Key: Love your brain; Love yourself; You are amazing

15

⸙

27 September 2021: FFS, I'm Sick Of Feeling Dizzy!

FFS. I'm sick of feeling Dizzy!

This constant nausea and topsy-turviness started when the Stoke hit on Sept 11, 2021, and it hasn't gone away. I hate it!

Every moment of every day is an opportunity to surrender to this feeling and affirm my future state of stability and "solidness"

I know that the more I pay attention to the Dizziness, the more it gains strength, that's how the law of attraction works right? We can attract what we don't want just as well as what we do want... in fact we can do that easily, for we practice attention on what we don't want far easier than what we do want and so

> *we get more of what we don't want!*
> *Simple right? Yeah in theory.*
> *But the challenge is rising above the current reality and assuming the feeling of the future state. That is the secret to all deliberate creation and I need to practice this now more than ever!*

One of the major changes in my body (head) has been the constant feeling of dizziness. As I write this on 24 February 2022, I recall this post from 27 September 2021 written from my hospital bed. The dizziness was intense and it's still with me today, but somehow different.

The difference is a result of healing. Not everything heals so quickly. I have a deeper knowing that the dizziness will eventually stop and that one day my former balanced state will return. Until then, I'll continue with the exercises that help build the neurology that will replace damaged brain tissue from the stroke of 11 September 2021.

On that day on the 27th, I was sick and tired of the dizziness; I'd had enough of it on that day.

However, the opportunity to surrender and affirm my future desired state is always available to me. The trick is to take that opportunity. I can't lie, on some days that is a hard choice to make. Affirming the desired future state when the current reality is far from that desired future state can be incredibly hard.

I suppose the answer is self-belief and faith.

I am a firm believer in the laws of the universe; in this case the law of attraction.

We live on our earthly plane subject to the law of cause and effect and in that sense, I realise that I can cause the effect on my future reality if I choose to do so. I can also attract whatever I am a vibrational match with.

I also believe my thoughts become things. This is all tied up together in my worldview; the law of cause and effect; the law of attraction; and the power of thought can all work for me to build a future desired state. But the choice is always mine; I always have free will to choose.

Transformation Key: You are always at choice with your thoughts; Think about your future positive outcome

16

27 September 2021: ...And Just Like That...

I was discharged.

My determination; the continued support from Claire; the amazing work of my physiotherapy team; the care I'd received from the nursing staff; and the medical expertise I'd received from the doctors and consultants, all combined with my vision and thoughts of returning home, had produced this result. Everything had worked together to bring me the outcome that I had desired when I was in the hospital. I was now ready to go home to continue my recovery surrounded by my family.

Home - The Annex

17

27 September 2021: ...And We're Home!!!

...and we're home!!!

Into the arms of my love Claire Chapman who has made the transition from hospital to home so smooth and seamless. Stress-free and perfect

The overwhelming feeling is that the silence is deafening, the peace and quiet is amazing. I'm so grateful for all the amazing NHS staff who looked after me but now that gratitude flows towards Claire and Roger Gough and Anita Gough for swapping homes to allow me to recuperate in safety and enjoy ground-level living

Thank you to all these incredible people and to all the wishes of love and support from FB friends across the world.

Feeling the love

I was delighted to go home. It was like winning first prize! Claire was an angel and paid so much attention to making my transition from hospital to home so smooth and peaceful.

Claire's parents Anita and Roger live next door to us. Whilst we occupy the primary house, Anita and Roger live in a gorgeous single-story annexe. They were both away in their motorhome so they kindly allowed me to stay there when I came out of hospital.

It was an ideal setting; everything was on a single story so I didn't have to cope with stairs.

I recall the actual journey home travelling in our Transporter. I was so weak and cold; there was an Autumn chill in the air so I was pleased with the blankets in the car as we left the hospital. I couldn't believe I was heading home; Really? Now? Already?

What next?

When we got home I went straight into the annex. Claire settled me in. I settled into Roger's recliner chair and Claire gave me one of our cosy blankets. She made sure I had everything I needed and then left me to mentally settle in. I slept deeply.

Transformation Key: Mentally celebrate all the wins no matter how big or small

18

28 September 2021: Routines Are Thrown In The Air!

Routines are thrown into the air!

What was normal is now far from normal!

All we can do is surrender to what is and somehow carve a path of healing on our way.

Claire Chapman, you are an absolute gem thank you so much for everything.

I notice how little things mean so much to me. The little things that make a situation perfect or the little things that can make a situation so frustrating. Working with Claire, she gets the balance just right, when to make it perfect and when to stop it getting frustrating.

> *As we journey through this recovery together we will discover new details that fall into these categories: that fine line between perfect and frustrating*
> *Claire, I love you so much, thank you for your patience, care and understanding*

Life at home recovering from a stroke had now started. Claire was incredible. Her level of care and attention was perfect. I remember thinking how (within time) I didn't want Claire to be my carer. I remember thinking, "No, Claire is my fiance, not my carer. I will be able to care for myself one day without any form of caring dependency on Claire."

But that level of independence would have to wait for now. In that period, Claire cared for me so much. She organised everything in my world. I could manage my toilet and washing but everything else was down to Claire. Wow, that is a lot!! Thank you Claire xxx

Transformation Key: Build a positive mindset

19

29 September 2021: Afraid But Determined

Afraid but determined.

I'm determined to let my body heal with grace and patience but I have to admit I have moments when I'm scared for the future.

3 weeks ago I was working on a new service for the Enterprise IT industry, today, that customer had to move with another supplier, and my ability to expand on the former work is limited by my lack of energy. Everything makes me so tired

I suppose the answer is to be kind to myself

Part 2:

Claire popped in and asked "Do you want to do some walking? The sun is out and it's beautiful"

Wow, just what I needed. I was falling into a slump; I was scared for the future; I was feeling sorry for myself.

> *She is so understanding. So empathetic; so caring.*
>
> *So I went outside and walked up and down the road, then sat in the sun, feeling the warmth on my face. Wow, instant mood changer.*
>
> *And then Gemma Tulett rocked up with homemade cottage pie for us all - yummy- thank you Gem!!*
>
> *Life is good - no matter how shit I had thought it was 60 mins earlier*

Throughout this entire recovery, I have had moments when I've been scared for the future. The overwhelming sense of uncertainty is something that I've had to reconcile.

I've lived with uncertainty many times before and somehow I've been able to define a more stable near-term outcome or certain outlook.

In the early part of 2021 and then leading up to the stroke, I had been working with a business partner to secure a fairly large contract with a global organisation that required my help. We had just secured the initial order and I was about to start the work with an assessment of their global IT Service Management capabilities. Ironically, I was due to start work on their assessment on Monday, September 13 2021, which was the Monday following the weekend of the stroke. Unsurprisingly, I couldn't continue with the assessment, and someone else had to be assigned to the customer instead of me. I also was doing some sub-contract software development/configuration work for another client. Both of these contracts, the global IT assessment and the software configuration work were lost. They combined to yield revenues of about £30,000 which left a gaping hole in the future family budget and ability to cover living expenses; and 3 months later, we would have Christmas. Yes, I was feeling very uncertain about the future.

Some incredible moments helped relieve some of that uncertainty. Claire was able to secure some new clients in her business and friends within our network marketing community pulled together to send us almost $5000 of BTC (bitcoin). These were amazing moments and the generosity of our networking friends was incredible and something I'll never forget. However, the bigger picture and financial concerns didn't go away.

On most days, I was too tired to be concerned. In hindsight, I think that was probably a good thing. I was too tired to do anything about the situation anyway, so I had no choice but to surrender the entire situation and hand it all over to God.

There were and still are many days when nothing makes any sense. It would be so very easy to have a horrible meltdown about the situation but that would not help. As a great believer in the Law of Attraction, I believe that we attract who/what we are. In that sense, I believe that if I were to worry and create fear in my body about any situation, then I am more likely to attract that situation into my reality, in other words, I would attract into my life, the very thing that I don't want.

My normal approach to this type of situation would have been to think positively and create opportunities for myself so I could provide service to someone and create an income stream. On this occasion and given the mess I was in because of the stroke, those previous routes to resolution were not available to me; oh no!!

All I had to do at this stage was focus on my physical recovery. I was living in the annex and Claire would leave me to myself for most of the day. She would arrange things for me and pop over to check I was ok but by and large, she would ensure I was safe and ok and then leave me to it; it worked well, and the balance between care and pushing me was perfect.

The very first couple of times of walking outside were quite unnerving. Claire would come over and ask, "Do you want to do some walking? The sun is out and it's beautiful." I love waking especially in the sunshine; I think there's nothing more spiritually uplifting. But I was nervous. My walking was still so unsteady; and unbalanced and I walked (or shuffled) very tentatively. I felt like a toddler taking his first steps, yet I was a 53-year-old man who had previously enjoyed sports and led an active lifestyle; what had happened to me? It was upsetting.

I would walk as much as I could in the sun. I suppose in the first days of walking outside I might have walked, or more like shuffled, about 50 yards. I then extended the journey a little more the next day and so on. Each day I was determined to walk a little further than previously.

After walking on those late summer days I would rest and sit in the warm sun. The sun is a brilliant antidote for feeling low; it can't be beaten in my opinion.

We had so much help being extended to our family from friends and neighbours, Gemma made us cottage pie and Lins (from the rugby club) made us lasagna on several occasions. Those meals were so welcome. It meant that Claire didn't have to worry about feeding the family on those occasions; which was a very welcome relief for her.

It was in those moments of sitting in the sun after a walk and getting homemade meals delivered by friends, that despite all the hardship, life felt good again, even if it was just for that brief moment.

Transformation Key: Accept help with gratitude and love

20

❦

3 October 2021: Patients and Patience

I wonder if the reason we call people in health recovery, patients, is because they have to have so much patience?!

OMG, I felt the need for patience myself this week. Claire who has so much patience with me, has repeatedly said that this is an injury like any other (sort of like a broken leg that needs to be repaired, except this is an injured brain) whereas I've had a lot of moments of seeing this as something far more permanent

Those are two very different perspectives and they have very different levels of impact on one's mental well-being.

This past week can be summed up as mentally challenging

On the upside I've been home, I've walked outside, I've travelled up/down the stairs, I've allowed healing through sleep, I've had visits from Physio Therapy, I've received incredible levels of care and compassion for which I'm incredibly grateful, I've watched loads of documentaries, football and golf on the TV which I wouldn't normally watch.

On the downside, I've been constantly feeling sick and dizzy

I've been awake at night with constipation (which I've overcome now phew)

I've fallen into a spell of depression by thinking this was permanent.

It's interesting to write this post, as the first list is far greater than the second list . When I ask myself why do I write these posts?

I realise that the answer is I write them for me. It's a journal of reflection that allows me to see that this past week hasn't been mentally challenging at all, but much more positive and full of upside. It's only been mentally challenging if I say it has.

Something is whatever we say it is!!!

It is whatever meaning we attach to it!!!

If we say something is hard then it's hard! If it's easy then it's easy!

If we say something is permanent then that's probably the outcome, if something is temporary then it will pass.

Wow, I'm going to sit with these words this afternoon as I look out of my window onto the garden and fields beyond. Nature is beautiful, abundant and forever changing.

Nothing is forever, everything is temporary

Here's to next week and the changes that it will bring.

Onwards and upwards!!

This was the moment that the concept of continuous transformation hit me. It was also the moment when I realised that having patience was going to be something that I needed to master, and I'd need to master it pretty damn soon.

In my former working world, transformation was always being discussed, it was always the topic of blogs and articles in the business IT sense.

Now here I was, right in the centre of my real-life transformation drama. It was becoming more obvious to me that this transformation was going to take time so I had to be very patient.

As I thought about this, it made me think about the word patient. In the English language we generally use the word to represent two things:

1. Being a patient in a healthcare system. I was a patient in that sense and had been since 12 September 2021
2. Showing or demonstrating patience whilst in the process of waiting for an outcome.

To achieve a successful and strong recovery, it became increasingly obvious to me that I would have to have great patience with myself and my situation.

As I considered the words patients and patience, it brought a smile to my face; the irony and humour were not lost on me so that aspect of my brain and character was all still functioning. Claire had already said to me that to heal my brain injury it would be like healing a broken leg. There is some truth in that similarity I suppose but as I later found out, an injury to the brain is much more profound than an injured limb. As the central process unit (CPU) for the entire body, the brain is responsible for the correct function of everything in one's reality, and when it's not working correctly the effects can be extreme.

I started to consider my situation and assessed each moment as either a positive or negative experience. This was not a deliberate strategy on my part, it just happened that way; things were either good or bad. As I considered specific events or circumstances that occurred during the days of early October, I started to become very grateful for the small positives that happened. The vastness of the overall negative situation was too much to bear, so I chose to focus on the small positives instead. Walking outside, walking up and down the stairs in our family home, healing through sleep, visits from physiotherapists, care from Claire, and time to watch sports on the TV were all examples of things I could be grateful for; these were opportunities to take as positive if I chose to.

The symptoms of my situation were coming into my awareness as well. These symptoms were categorised as negative in my psyche at that time. The continuous dizziness and nausea were starting to get me down; it seemed endless. Another symptom of being immobilised was an increasing level of constipation. I never realised how constipation could affect someone. Luckily, and apologies for the detail here, I have always been blessed with a regular constitution; my first activity of the day is my early morning poo! Yep, I never thought I'd ever write that but there we go, it's out there now (lol). When I was so immobile, my bowls seemed to bung up. I was drinking as much water as I could but I was still becoming dehydrated and combined with the lack of physical movement, the overall effect was constipation. It was amazing how these things contributed to my overall well-being. Being constipated made me feel... well er shit I suppose. There's another irony right there. The lack of or inability to crap, made me feel crap. I'm sorry if that seems a bit crude or unnecessary but it's true. Being constipated became a thing. I hated it. I remember being so relieved when the constipation eased. I was so grateful when my ability to go to the toilet returned to normal. I don't ever take going for a poo for granted ever again; I'm so grateful for a healthy digestion, gut and bowl system.

I started to question myself and why I wrote the social media posts. I recalled listening to an amazing coach who had coached Claire for a while. I recalled her saying that a particular platform has a feature called memories and it is an amazing way of looking back over one's life and seeing progress. So in that sense, in that moment I realised that I wrote the posts primarily for me. I was using that platform feature as a diary. If someone else liked them then great, in my mind that was a bonus. I later discovered that not only did people like them, they found them inspiring and in some cases, the posts helped others with stroke. I had no idea of the power of my words. When I found out that I'd been able to help other stroke survivors with my words, I was so pleased and felt a huge feeling of love I'd never felt before; it was a love for strangers; a love and a deep sense of compassion for others that I'd never felt before.

Another thing that started to come into my reality was a sense of perspective. I've always thought that Claire is a master at perspective; she has this incredible way of looking at a situation from multiple dimensions and perspectives that allows her to witness the situation rather than play the central role in the drama; It's a brilliant gift that she teaches others.

So in early October and with Claire's help, I also started to appreciate the perspective. I started to become a witness to my emotions and feelings. I found it much easier to cope with the effects of the stroke and the situation that I found myself in by being the witness rather than the central character, even though I was that central character. As I started to understand my situation a bit more, I realised that my posts also provided me with a point of reflection. It was that reflection that then led to an enhanced perspective and in the way it then led to a greater sense of gratitude for what was going well in my life.

I suppose this period was a turning point for me. It was just over 3 weeks since the stroke and I realised that my life was never going to be the same again. I had a choice. I could mourn for the death of my former life or I could look forward to the new life that was coming; in other words, I could rebuild my life; it was my choice which path I would now take.

I could give up and become the victim and blame the world for my predicament or I could take the opportunity to start over. I thought to myself, "Wow, how many people get that opportunity?" I had survived the stroke; I hadn't been a victim of stroke; it was going to be my gift. Yes, things would be different; that was obvious; I would have to adapt and learn new ways of doing things and I didn't know what those things would be until I realised at the moment; but that's exciting in a way; there's always something to learn; always something to discover; it's a bit like being a young child on the pathway of discovery all over again.

As I started to reflect more, I had to decide if I was going to see the effects of stroke as permanent damage or something that would pass. I decided that this would all pass. If I looked at the stroke as permanent damage, it would be too easy to fall into a depressed state and I hadn't survived just to become depressed. I understood that things would not be normal, but then what the heck is normal anyway!? Who gets to decide what's normal? My 'new normal' might be different from my 'old normal', which would be ok. I was alive! The journey was onward and upwards and one of continuous discovery and change. Wow, bring it on!

Transformation Key: Nothing is permanent; Everything is temporary.

21

6 October 2021: Kindness - Support - Love - Generosity

Kindness - Support - Love - Generosity
These are the keywords that I/we have felt these past 2 weeks since I left hospital to continue my recovery at home.
Messages of support, Meals cooked for us, Bitcoin dropping into our wallet from what seems like "out of the sky"!
Every day, Claire tirelessly inspires me to take action to speed my recovery (her love is limitless). The love and support that I/ we have received has been overwhelming.
Words cannot describe the feeling of love and appreciation in my heart for everyone giving to us/me so generously and unconditionally... thank you all so so much

The overwhelming spirit of kindness and love carries me through the dark days giving me hope for now and the future.
Without hope there is nothing and this outpouring of love and support delivers hope in bucket loads!!
Thank you thank you thank you

The messages and comments on my social media posts were so supportive and full of love; it was so generous of people to take the time to read my posts and then comment; I was overwhelmed.

As mentioned before, we had been given meals; bitcoin had been sent to us; we had witnessed a very generous side to the human condition, it was lovely and something I will never forget.

Claire was a massive source of inspiration for me. Her love and care would make me take the actions that I needed to do if I was going to rebuild myself.

This was a time when I felt so much love from different people and it made a difference that helped carry me through and encouraged me to not dwell during the darker moments.

Transformation Key: Feel the love flowing to you

22

8 October 2021: There will be Good Days and Not So Good Days

There will be Good Days and Not So Good Days

Yesterday I had a good day. A lot of things made sense, my energy was up and I felt like progress was being made.

Today, not so much. I'm completely exhausted and keep falling asleep. Unable to even focus or concentrate on tasks.

The words that come forth are to be kind to myself, forgiveness and peace, and acceptance of what is. Don't beat myself up or come down on myself, some days won't be as good as others, and that's ok. It is what it is!

Recovery is a strange beast, you're up then you're down.

Yesterday when I was up I seemed to achieve so much:

I had a great conversation with my elder brother, Phil, who had a similar stroke about 3 years ago. Speaking with Phil provides me with hope as he has made a fantastic recovery. We spoke of many things but he told me about how he had enjoyed building Lego Technic models during his recovery. This lit me up So I ordered a Ducati Panigale V4R which has been delivered today

Following a visit from Physio Therapy (yesterday) my understanding of brain plasticity and neural pathway recovery increased which helped with my understanding of what I'm going through....it's fascinating stuff!

I wrote several chapters (small) of my book capturing my thoughts and feelings all about this crazy journey - if it can help someone else then great! All good positive stuff.

Today has been nothing but sleep and rest. But after yesterday's understanding, I'm ok with that. The poor old brain is exhausted

Forming new neural networks is bloody hard work. What I used to do second nature is no longer there! But the brain is so advanced that it will carve out new pathways to achieve the same outcome ... wow wow wow! But as I'm doing so the brain also recognises that these new pathways are unknown and unfamiliar so it sends other signals to my body to reject this new idea (pathway), such as making me feel sick. So my brain is having a battle with itself- holy shit, no wonder I'm so knackered!!!

So I'm signing off now as writing this post has made me even more tired

> *Let's hope I can start building this model later, but if not there's always tomorrow, there's no rush*

Throughout my recovery, I've had both good days and bad days. I became aware of this duality in early October 2021. It has continued to this day; good days and not-so-good days.

I no longer use negative language if I can help it, so instead of saying bad days, I just state them as "not so good" days. Another language shift I've had to make is around brain injury. I got into the habit of describing the damage in my brain and Claire made me aware of how often I'd speak of brain damage so I've shifted that to speak about damage repair or brain rebuilding.

The idea of these shifts is very simple. The power of the word is immense. If I say my brain is damaged or I have bad days, I'll create more of that in reality. If I think those thoughts, and then worse, speak them out loud, then I am affirming that those conditions are true. God/Source Energy/The Universe responds in such a way that those conditions are repeated over and over and the condition becomes my reality.

So, by changing my thoughts and words, I can create a different reality. Thinking and speaking of rebuilding my brain and "not so good" days is like playing tricks with the universe and making the universe bend to my will. Do I control the universe? Well in a sense, yes, I can control my universe if I want to. As you do with yours! We all create our reality based on our thoughts, feelings, conditions, perspectives and pattern-ing. In that sense, we all create our version of the universe, and given that we are all made from the very same particles and substances of the physical universe (stardust is another way of looking at it) we are intrinsically linked to and fully part of the universe whilst simultaneously creating our universe with our version of reality in any given moment.

One of the first people I spoke to was my brother, Phil. Phil also had a brain haemorrhage (stroke) a number a few years ago. Yes, two brothers in the same family. Unlucky right!? We were both of similar ages when the bleeds occurred; early 50s. Like anyone who's had a stroke, his experience was unique to him. But there were similarities and being able to speak to someone (especially a surviving family member) helped me a great deal.

During one such conversation, Phil told me how he had built several Lego Technics models during his recovery. I was interested in this approach and it seemed like it could be fun whilst also beneficial to my recovery. He continued to recommend a particular model; the Ducati Panigale V4R motorcycle. We both share an interest in motorcycles and motorcycling, so I went ahead and ordered one online. I was excited to take delivery of the model and was looking forward to getting started and building it. As I write this almost 5 months later, it still isn't finished. I work on it for a while and then stop for weeks on end. It will be finished at some point, I'm sure.

I was also getting several visits from the local physiotherapy team, also known as the Wiltshire Early Support Discharge (ESD) team. Every member of that team was brilliant. Some were focused on my core strength; I recall Lara (who led the team) helped me with several exercises to help me with my core strength and balance. Another physiotherapist, Kate, helped me with fine motor skills and working through the dizziness and nausea. I recall her first visit with me. She sat with me and explained neuroplasticity to me. It was a wonderful explanation that helped me understand what had happened as a result of the stroke and helped me understand how my brain was recovering.

As a result of that explanation, I was able to understand that the specific area of my brain that was flooded with blood from the bleed, would never repair itself, but the brain would build new neural pathways to re-establish the damaged connections. I found this information fascinating. Furthermore, as the brain builds new pathways it simultaneously sends messages to the body to stop that rebuilding from happening. This sounds strange so let me explain what I mean.

The brain controls everything and it has an amazing capacity to rebuild and expand itself (as well as shrink). My brain was injured by the bleeding, so it wanted to repair itself, but at the same time it didn't like the stress of rebuilding so it would send messages to other parts of my body to stop me from doing whatever it was I was doing that caused it stress. The messages were intended to make me stop and I would feel nauseous and dizzy, although a lot of the dizziness was also caused by the bleed being in the cerebellum which controls the balance in the body, so that neurology had been destroyed.

I find all this such an interesting thing; the brain gets injured and neurology gets damaged so that the brain then rebuilds the neurology but in the process, it doesn't like the rebuilding process so it attempts to stop that from happening by creating upset in the body to force the human to stop whatever it is doing to help rebuild the neurology.

Everything that was happening to me was starting to make sense to me. Up to that point, I had the impression that the blood would disperse from the affected area of my brain and the damaged brain tissue would repair itself. I'm not a medical expert or a trained neurologist so please don't read this as expert advice but having the understanding that my brain was attempting to rebuild and construct brand-new neurology to replace the damaged tissue made perfect sense to me. I imagined that the main neural routes that had been established over decades of my human experience were now gone and wouldn't be repaired, they were being replaced. New routes were being established so that communication in the brain could take place again.

I thought of a metaphor based on the road system and the UK motorway network. The metaphor went something like this:

The previous neurology and communication were like travelling from Swindon (my nearest major town) to London via the M4 Motorway, but imagine that the M4 gets damaged and needs to close and so travelling to London has to be established via an alternative or even new routes. These new routes might involve travelling through fields, streams and hedges and it would be tough work. It would be difficult to establish the new routes, not just to travel once, but to establish the routes in such a way that they were reliable, consistent, fast and repeatable. Not only would this be hard work but there would be resistance and protests about the creation of these new routes and all the while the existing M4 route remained closed. Eventually, the new routes would be established even though the existing M4 route remained closed (forever). It's a rather crude analogy and metaphor but it made sense to my simplistic view of the situation.

These discoveries were fascinating to me and I got to enjoy the process of recovery, albeit the enjoyment was somewhat limited.

On other days the recovery would be exhausting, especially in the early weeks. If I had done some physio, had a conversation or just managed a very short walk I then just wanted to sleep.

I realised that my poor brain was simply tired. All the work it was doing was making my brain dog-tired. I never knew brain fatigue would be such a thing. It's awful. So I would sleep and on some days (not many) that was all I wanted to do from the moment I woke in the morning. It was on those sorts of days that I would notice that I felt quite low. Those were the "not-so-good days. When I felt low the emotions of sadness, frustration and anger would rise and it was then that I discovered my ability to forgive myself.

Transformation Key: Learn and understand how the brain and body transform to help create your reality.

23

9 October 2021: "What doesn't kill you, makes you stronger."

"What doesn't kill you, makes you stronger."

Wise words indeed. In a conversation with my brother, Phil, on Thursday morning, he used this well-known phrase.

4 weeks ago today I had a haemorrhagic stroke (bleed in the brain) that could have easily killed me. But it didn't and here I am at home on the slow road of recovery…. I'm learning how to be a patient patient…not easy for me I can tell you!!!

Earlier this week, my gorgeous eldest daughter Bryony and her boyfriend Jack had arranged for a lovely gift to be delivered which included the book, "The Obstacle Is The Way", by Ryan Holiday. I was touched as they live in Bondi, New South Wales,

Aus. In a land far far far away. Wasn't that in Shrek?

This afternoon I've been reading a lot, especially this book and at almost midpoint was the phrase, "What doesn't kill you, makes you stronger".

God delivers messages in mysterious ways that always make me smile.

Things might appear difficult to me now but compared to near death 4 weeks ago, my progress is remarkable!!! I feel blessed with every new day.

Today I sat in the sunshine in the garden while the boys mowed the grass (great job boys!!), I trimmed my beard which had become spikey and uncomfortable in recent days, Claire cut my hair and I had a shower (to get rid of any loose hairs).

All in all quite a progressive morning with a lot more in there as well I know that "this too shall pass"

I'm hearing so many stories of similar stroke cases where full recoveries have occurred and even better outcomes than pre-stroke in some cases.

My intention is that this will be my story, I will come back stronger, wiser, more patient, with greater love, more grace and forgiveness, more tolerant, more understanding, more generous and giving with my time and energy, more helpful, my intention is to be a better man with more to give to others.

"What doesn't kill you makes you stronger" will be a phrase carved into my psyche forever a life motto perhaps. New tattoo maybe who knows but definitely wise words to live by.

With love

I love the way that God communicates with us. We often put these down as coincidences, but I prefer to look beyond what we generally call coincidence, serendipity, intuition and gut feel, I prefer to smile and say,

"OK God, I hear and see you. Thanks for the message".

These types of events happen often to me, and I think they do for most people. God speaks to us in mysterious ways. This happened during the latter part of the week of October 3-10, 2021.

The phrase, "What doesn't kill you makes you stronger," was coming through from several sources. As I write this now (almost 5 months later), I am reminded of the phrase again and it still carries a significance after that passage of time.

Phil had visited on the Thursday morning of that week in October 2021 and then I was reading a chapter from a book sent to me by my eldest daughter, Bryony and her boyfriend Jack, on the following Saturday. Both Phil and the book gave me the message within that phrase. Coincidence? Maybe, or maybe not. I don't know. But I took it as a message; a message of hope and resilience to keep going and dig deep throughout the recovery

I felt my connection with God getting stronger. The messages of fortitude were coming through thick and fast, and I felt a growing sense of determination rising within me. I also had an overwhelming sense of gratitude for just being alive and

I felt that I wanted to nurture qualities in me that needed more of both my attention and intention.

I knew that the new version of me was going to have to have more love, more grace, more forgiveness, more tolerance, and be more generous with my time and energy. I've had several messages from former work colleagues over these past 6 months and I've been pleased by how many people and lives I've positively influenced over my former years before the stroke. As a result of those messages, I don't feel that these are qualities that were necessarily missing in my old self but it would do no harm at all to hone, tune and double-down on these qualities for my future self.

Transformation Key: Be grateful for what you have, and don't dwell on lack or loss.

24

❦

13 October 2021:
Stepping Outside

Stepping Outside

.... is going to be a daily discipline within this recovery.

I've always loved walking in the countryside and we are blessed to live in the countryside so walking up and down the lane is such great therapy.

As I walked alone up the lane I could hear the sound of birds. Crows "cawing" in the distance. In flocks, as they flew over the fields swooping low to brush the field and then up high calling to one another... it was an amazing sound and the experience was breathtaking.

Although fairly mundane for a country walk, I've missed these moments more than I realised.

I was reminded of my childhood and the village setting where I lived with my family. I would watch and listen to the crows high up in the trees on the old castle mound leading to the village's 10th-century church. Those crows seemed to call stories going back over those hundreds of years, back to when the castle was solid and thriving. Tales of ancient Cotswold village life which according to historical records was anything but quaint.

I cherish these opportunities to step outside as they spark my imagination, allow me to breathe in the fresh air, they allow me a moment of "normality" that is not beset with continuous feelings of travel sickness.

These moments to wander outside are to become a daily habit for me. I love them

I'm not entirely sure of the physical benefits (although I am sure there are many), mentally, they are a gift from god to be cherished

By mid-October, 2021, I was walking alone outside. Considering that only the month before I was unable to walk at all, the progress was going well. Once I started to walk outside, it became a regular daily habit that I cherished.

Walking was great physiotherapy and even better for my mental health. It was the time of year when Autumn was drawing in, there was a chill in the air but it was predominantly dry. I've always enjoyed walking in the countryside, but during my recovery, walking outside was a huge boost for me, both physically and mentally. One of the aspects of walking in the countryside that truly lights up my soul is the sound of the birds. I cannot claim to be a birdsong expert, but since spending time taking daily walks in my local area I can now distinguish the sound of buzzards, blackbirds, robins, sparrows, skylarks, crows and wood pigeons. I don't know what it is about birdsong, and particularly the sound of buzzards and skylarks seems to have a deeper place in my heart, but I have an overwhelming sense of peace wash over me when I'm walking alone in the countryside and I hear those beautiful calls and songs.

I am so grateful for the local area where I live. The countryside is literally on the doorstep. I think being able to breathe in the fresh air, stretch my legs outside and take in the beauty of nature has contributed greatly to my recovery and transformation.

Transformation Key: Get outside in nature, breathe in the fresh air; listen to the birds; and feel the connection with Mother Earth.

25

14 October 2021: FFS Back In Hospital Again!! Nooooo!

FFS Back in the hospital again!! Noooooo!

Had severe chest pains this evening and my blood pressure spiked (can't remember the reading now).

Claire called 999 but the ambulance service is completely overwhelmed at the moment- don't bother calling for an ambulance you'll probably not get one!

So Claire drove me up to Swindon Great Western Hospital A&E (it's so busy!!) and now here I am.... waiting for results from ECG and blood tests... feeling well and truly crap.

On the upside, at least the chest pains have stopped

It might not all be smooth sailing (as they say), but that is ok. At the time it does feel crap, and again, that is ok. If it feels crap, then it feels crap. The secret to handling the dips is to not attach any meaning to it. It would be very easy for me to attach the meaning of "I'm having another stroke", or "My recovery is failing", or "I'm dying" to an event like this, and I can't deny it, those thoughts did flash through my mind but only for a split-second. The overarching thought was "Damn, this is annoying" and then I moved on and thought about something else pretty quickly.

I recall having a feeling of frustration mixed with relief. The pain in my chest had eased before I'd arrived in the hospital and I was still alive; no heart attack; no stroke (as far as I could tell) and now, no more chest pain, so huge relief in that sense, but I was also frustrated with sitting around in the A&E department which was very busy. I ended up waiting there for hours while the tests that they had run were checked out by a doctor.

I think about this now one year later (October 2022). To even have an ounce of frustration seems ridiculous to me now. I suppose that is a sign of how far I have grown in that year. I mean, think about it, how could I have any frustration with the situation when the chest pains had stopped, there was no heart attack and I wasn't having another stroke? Frustrated at what exactly? As I sit here writing about that event one year on, I have nothing but immense gratitude in my body. I think we're so quick to judge a situation as good or bad and it just is and the experience is nothing but an experience.

When I did eventually see a doctor, I was hugely relieved to be told that everything was fine and I could go home again. Yes! In my imagination, I punched the air in celebration.

Transformation Key: Try not to judge a situation as either good or bad, it is just an experience and nothing more. Judging a situation just causes unnecessary unease in the body.

26

14 October 2021: I'm Home Again!

I'm home again!!! whoopee!!! I've never loved my own bed quite so much.

The poor NHS emergency services are at breaking point, it's very sad to see and even worse to experience.

The ambulance service is almost non-existent with telephone call queues like a utility call centre. The ETA for an ambulance is 3-4 hours when you do finally speak to a human being.

The Emergency Dept is unbelievably busy...So many people need help!!

The triage try their best to stem the tide but they become stressed and lose their duty of care for the sick and frightened.

The doctors can't cope with the demand to assess the results of blood tests and ECG, X-rays etc

That leaves patients waiting in the waiting areas while more and more people flood through the doors!

It never stops!

Last night, I saw sports injuries, pregnant ladies, COVID cases, and stroke cases, I had heart concerns on top of the stroke, the variety of conditions was unbelievable..and we all needed help. Not one of us wanted to be there out of choice.

So, thank you God for :

Giving me the all-clear from any heart abnormalities

Giving me a wonderful caring Claire Chapman who can balance so much on her plate including fetching me home at 5 a.m. and giving me a comfortable bed in which to rest and catch up on lost sleep.

Giving me the countryside setting in which to continue my recovery (thank you Roger and Anita Gough for your wonderful home)

Surrounding me with love and support

God, please bless those in NHS A&E.

I was so relieved to be home again. Although my visit to the A&E department was relatively short (about 7 hours), I was so grateful to be back home.

I recall a moment when a lady pushed her husband into the A&E dept reception area in a wheelchair. He could barely breathe and looked very ill. I immediately thought Covid. Sure enough, they were quickly ushered towards a dedicated entrance for Covid cases but of course, it was too late, he had been in the reception area where I was sitting.

"Oh no, not Covid as well, no thank you, God, please protect me", I thought to myself. I was a sitting duck so all I could do was think about my well-being and then thoroughly wash my hands as soon as I was able to. I thought to myself that if I thought I was going to catch COVID-19 then I probably would, so I maintained an approach of protection for myself with my positive thinking and hygiene actions (thorough hand washing etc.) I also wrapped myself within an energetic bubble of protection. To some people, this may sound silly, but at that moment when I was potentially exposed to Covid, I couldn't do anything else, I was literately sat in a chair unable to move out of the way, so I had to energetically assume that I was protected and nothing (not even Covid) was going to get me.

It worked, I didn't catch Covid.

I witnessed an Emergency Health Service creaking during that evening. The demand was relentless. It was an extremely stressful place to be. I found it interesting how two nurses doing the same job could provide such different levels of care.

The scenario was this: They were both working within the Triage function of the Emergency department. They were both doing the same job with the same facilities with the same demand of patient after patient, both nurses were the same except for the colour of their uniform (so rank was different). One nurse was lovely. She was caring; considerate;

compassionate; she took her time to listen; she acted on the concerns of patients as best she could. The other was the complete opposite and did not demonstrate any of those qualities. At first, I judged the second nurse for her abruptness and intolerance, but later after I'd understood my invalid judgement, I realised that there might have been a whole host of additional reasons behind her behaviour. I realised that I could only witness what I could witness, I didn't know anything. There could have been any number of things bothering her; the list is potentially countless. This was quite a profound moment for me. My former self might have immediately judged the second nurse, but the newer version of me was starting to understand perspective and it was evident that I was also making a concerted effort to drop my judgement; maybe it was starting to be effective.

The A&E Department was heaving and no one wanted to be there; not one patient had made the choice to spend the evening and night in the A&E department, but there we all were: Stroke Survivors (me), Covid patients, pregnant ladies, people with sports injuries, the patients and a variety of ill-health conditions that went on and on, and the nursing staff kept working through the demand, patiently and diligently.

When I returned home I had time to reflect on my experience that evening and I practised some minutes of gratitude for everything that was good in my life and what was in contrast to the discomfort to the A&E department. Practicing gratitude was becoming a regular part of my life experience and it felt good. I found it a way of staying grounded in any given event or set of circumstances.

Transformation Key: Change your habits: Swap judgment for gratitude.

27

〰️

15 October 2021: Slowing down is the new Speeding Up

Slowing down is the new Speeding Up
This has to be my mantra for the week!
Today my physiotherapy session even took the form of Pilates.
My head/eye exercises have become gentle small movements and
my overall attitude towards life has now got to be "slow down".
I've realised that I have been a worrier. If there's something to
worry about then I'll worry about it!! I think I follow my mum
in that regard, she's the same, omg Thanks Mum (not!). In the
future, I'm going to have to learn how to build the pause button
into my life.
But all this can wait. Today, my elder brother, Phil, cycled over

to see me. That's an 80-mile round trip by someone who himself had a stroke 3 years ago!! He's as fit as a fiddle! We chatted loads, it was really great to see him and of course, we share a number of common experiences associated with stroke.

He gave some great advice. The worrying issue can wait, he said. Focus all your energy on getting well so that you have the energy to fight that battle when you're able to. Until then, don't worry about it!

Really good advice Thanks, Phil!

So with that, I'm signing off now to slow down and focus on getting well and nothing else.

By mid-October (just over one month into recovery) I realised that taking things at a slower pace was resulting in a healthier and more sustainable recovery of my life. "Rome wasn't built in a day" is a well-known saying and this applied to my recovery and more so, the creation of a new version of me.

As I've mentioned before, Phil, my elder brother, also survived a brain haemorrhage. His recovery over 3 years has been remarkable. So remarkable that he now rides his mountain road bike for great lengths (even completing a Lands-End to John O'Groats ride in 2022). The 80-mile round trip to come and visit me was a drop in the ocean for Phil. That gives you an indication of his recovery and self-determination. I guess it must run in the family. Stroke and self-determination that is!!

I have always been a worrier and worrying had not served

me very well at all. When I was initially in hospital after the stroke I had been subjected to countless tests to determine the source of my high blood pressure. The consultants could not find anything wrong with me physically so they attributed the high blood pressure and hypertension to stress. This made an awful lot of sense to me. I had been going through a lot of personal stress leading up to the stroke and throughout my entire life, I had carried far too much stress.

I was a persistent worrier. Everything made me worry. I was only consciously aware of certain stresses and worries; you know the normal things like money, children, family life, ex-relationships etc. But I think I had underlying worries and stresses too. I liked to have things in order; like the house; that was an underlying cause of stress for me. I like to keep a tidy house and have things in order. That is a very difficult thing to achieve with 8 of us and 2 dogs (sadly, we now just have one). So, I've subsequently learnt through this recovery process that I can't control or know everything; sometimes it's okay to just not know or if someone makes a mess then that's just okay and it will be cleared up later.

This is a huge shift for me. I used to want to be on top of these things as a form of protection for Claire; if I could protect her from this kind of thing then that was a good thing in my former worldview. It was during my recovery that I discovered that I couldn't control all these types of things; I would have to surrender control and just "let it go".

Life can be stressful, money, relationships, marriage, divorce, children, exams, bills, the job, the boss, career, course work, deadlines, to-do lists, goals, aspirations, fears, you name it, everything can make us stressed out.

In recent times, technology has also played a hand in creating an "always on or always available" culture affecting work/life balance and the dopamine hit from a reaction to your well-crafted and meaningful post on social media platforms. It all becomes a dopamine addiction and causes stress. Stress also comes in the form of work emails. I recall in my former marriage how as a senior leader, with staff working within my teams in both the UK and USA, I felt the need to be always available to respond to any emails. I always needed to immediately remove the pressure of the email sitting unread in my inbox; nothing could wait, which created a very unhealthy way of living. The odd thing is, I didn't expect the same behaviour from anyone else. I only had this expectation of myself. Looking back on it now, I had a very unhealthy way of treating myself and regretfully, my behaviour might have set the tone for others to behave the same without my conscious awareness. I think this is quite common in a lot of people. How we treat ourselves is not very nice; we're often not kind or compassionate with ourselves. Additionally, as a leader, we need to set an example for others.

Modern life is relentless and our brains are not designed for it. Our brains are designed to look for dangers; our brains are wired to protect us from creatures or enemies that wanted to kill us when we were hiding in our caves 40000 years ago. We're designed to respond to stress, but modern life turns that stress dial up the a constant maximum, so our brains and bodies are in an acute state of stress almost all the time which creates dis-ease in the body, such as Stroke, Cancer, Heart Dis-ease, Mental Health issues, the list can go on and on.

So with so much around to cause us to be stressed out, we need to ensure that we protect ourselves from further stress and recognise behaviours in ourselves that don't help.

Awareness of high blood pressure is key. It's a silent killer and doesn't show itself that often. Make sure you check your blood pressure. Don't obsess about it as that in itself could cause unnecessary stress and cause your blood pressure to become elevated. But be aware. Especially if there is a family history. Take it seriously and seek professional help and support. I now use an App to track my blood pressure, but I realise I should have done that before. Too little, too late in my case but I do it now to prevent any reoccurrence of brain haemorrhage or other issues linked to high blood pressure.

4 years ago in April 2017, I was taken to hospital with chest pains and it was found that I had high blood pressure. After a 24-hour spell in hospital, where I was intensely medicated to lower my blood pressure, I was prescribed medication to control it but at that time I thought I knew better and wanted to get myself off the medication as soon as I could. I used to monitor my blood pressure through a wrist-based monitor. The reading got down to the target 120/80 that my GP had set. Perfect! I was then able to sustain that level without daily medication, so I took myself off the medication.

Perhaps that wasn't such a smart move! I've subsequently discovered that the medical profession does not rate or recommend wrist-worn blood pressure monitors. Now I use a monitor with a cuff that goes above the elbow and I track the results manually in an App. The reason for tracking is to spot any trends or patterns in lifestyle and how those lifestyle influences impact my blood pressure levels. I've noticed that if I get anxious about anything then my blood pressure will start to rise.

The lesson in all this is that sometimes we don't always know better and there is a very good reason to heed the guidance and advice being offered to us, but maybe without obsessing over it. Since the stroke last September I've been prescribed far more medication than I was prescribed previously in 2017, which is somewhat ironic I suppose. Perhaps if I'd maintained the blood pressure medication and monitored it more diligently then maybe I wouldn't have experienced the haemorrhage at all!? I guess I'll never truly know. I'm pretty sure any medical professional would probably agree with that assessment but in all honesty, who truly knows?

I have included my blood pressure tracking results at the back of this book with tables and the corresponding charts showing monthly averages from September 2021 through to September 2022. I am pleased to say that throughout that time the blood pressure has steadily dropped.

I found the following note that I'd written around this time in my recovery. There's a critical message in there which is why I've decided to include it here.

As I looked at that diary entry from October 15 2021, I can remember that it was the third week into my recovery and I thought I had hit rock bottom, I had hit despair. I tried to remain positive with my responses to messages from people asking, "Hi Simon, how are you feeling?". I tried my best to answer as upbeat as I could, but inside I felt terrible, both physically and mentally.

I recall thinking that under the circumstances I shouldn't have felt like that. I was at home, Claire was amazing (as always), I was getting so much support and love, my recovery was progressing well and I was able to achieve more each day.

But as good, beautiful and amazing as all those things were, I couldn't see any of them at that time because despair had set in. I was blind to the goodness. I kept comparing how I was after the stroke with how I was before the stroke.

As I think about that now, that's a crazy thing to do, it's like comparing apples with oranges! It is pointless doing that type of comparison, although it's an inevitable reaction to the situation of course.

If you're reading this as someone recovering from a stroke, do yourself a big favour and don't do that comparison, it will severely affect your mental health and wellbeing, and very likely slow down any chance of recovery too.

To combat the despair, I managed to let the love flow to me rather than dwell on the loss of my former life.

I wrote a social media post and in it, I wrote how I was overwhelmed by the love and support that Claire and I had received since my return home. As I wrote that post my attitude changed in that moment. Instead of despair, I felt hope. I wrote these words:

"Words cannot describe the feeling of love and appreciation in my heart for everyone giving to us/me so generously and unconditionally..... thank you all so so much.

The overwhelming spirit of kindness and love carries me through the dark days giving me hope for now and the future.

Without hope there is nothing and this outpouring of love and support delivers hope in bucket loads!!

Thank you thank you thank you

Transformation Key: If you've experienced a setback in your life, don't compare your former life with your current situation; It's a pointless waste of energy that will hinder your transformation. Instead, use your energy to focus on love and your future self.

28

16 October 2021: Balance

BALANCE

Imagine you've just stepped off an intense fairground/theme park ride. You feel disoriented, everything is spinning, and you feel sick. You certainly can't eat anything, you need to sit down and wait for the awful feeling to stop before you can do anything.

Welcome to my world for the past 5 weeks.

I've always disliked fairground rides, especially in my adult life because that feeling is so awful, and now I'm having to contend with that all the time.

Even in bed lying down, I can shut my eyes and it can feel like I'm falling backwards, I have to open my eyes and in the darkness the feeling of falling stops, thank god!

Brain injury is so strange, it really is an inside job. People say to me that I look ok, but on the inside, I feel as rough as hell.

This morning I did my physio routine, which includes pretending to walk on a tightrope across the kitchen floor. One foot in front on the other. It's crazy, as simple as that sounds, I find it really difficult. I have to use the countertop for support and I'm only walking on the floor. Thank goodness I'm not actually on a real tightrope. If I was I'd be screwed! Let's just say I won't be joining the circus anytime soon

As you twist and turn throughout your day, be thankful for the amazing job your brain is doing that helps you always make sense of it all without feeling sick or disoriented. It's all so clever and we take it for granted.

I cannot wait for this to return to normal. That day I will have a huge party

The brain haemorrhage bled into the cerebellum area of my brain. My balance was severely affected. At first, my balance was so bad that I couldn't sit up or get up out of my hospital bed (I could only slide off and then crawl). Eventually, I noticed how things improved. It is now early March 2022 as I write this sentence, my balance is still unstable but the feeling has changed; it is now a kind of unbalanced as if I were trying to walk on the deck of a ship on the high seas, and the ship is leaning down towards the left side (port side). It certainly isn't fully repaired but all of the instant dizziness and accompanying nausea has passed. I've noticed that the new feeling, of standing on a leaning ship, is worse if I've spent a lot of time sitting down during the day. When I get up to walk, sometimes I find myself walking into doorframes or having to support myself on walls in the house as I walk around.

Walking outside makes a tremendous difference. My mental and physical state improves so much from a walk outside.

2 or 3 months ago the dizziness had changed into a sense of continuous falling. The only way I can describe it was that it felt like my brain was made of lead and it was too heavy for my skull. Throughout this entire journey the dizziness, falling, and unbalanced feeling have been alongside a fogginess that has clouded my thoughts. Today, March 2, 2022, I have got used to my poor short-term memory and my slightly impaired ability to do maths and construct sentences. Writing this book has taken a lot of effort, especially when I keep typing the wrong worms, I mean words.

I now incorporate yoga, pilates and press-ups into my daily routine. I do this routine twice a day. The routine is a non-negotiable for me; it must happen for me; both morning and night.

The training routine I've developed is an adaptation of a sun salutation routine incorporating yoga and pilates poses into a continuous flow which is then followed by my press-ups-based routine with more pilates-type poses and stretches. I have included the details of the routine at the back of the book so that you too can learn my flow.

This routine has helped me regain my strength, balance and posture. With the combination of plenty of walking out in nature, I find this has helped my recovery tremendously. If you are a stroke survivor and you would also like to try this routine then please do, however, it is advisable to consult a medical professional before doing so. If you wish to do this routine, you do so at entirely your own risk.

BTW: I didn't consult any medical professional before undertaking this twice-daily routine; but that was my decision which I felt was appropriate for me in my specific circumstances.

Transformation Key: Move your body. Do whatever you can. It might be small but anything is better than nothing. Your body is your vessel carrying you on your journey on planet Earth so nurture it and love it.

29

17 October 2021: It's So Good To Cry

It's so good to cry

Joy - Despair - Happiness - Sadness

It doesn't matter what emotion, the liberation from letting the tears flow is amazing

Some people turn to sad films to invoke the tears, for me it's music that sets me off.

This is by far my favourite piece of music, this entire album is a beautiful emotional journey. I listened today for the first time in over 12 months.

Wow, the tears flowed continuously.

Images of sadness to absolute ecstasy flowed through my mind, and memories from past and future experiences flashed through my imagination.

> *Beautiful. Joy. Dramatic. Powerful. Each bringing wave after wave of tears. Release. Relief. Liberation. Unlocking fear and sadness. No anger, just joy and optimism.*
> *This is what this album does for me. It's truly amazing.*
> *Wishing you a wonderful day*

The album I refer to in that post is Flow State by Above and Beyond. It's one of my favourites.

I think this day was a huge turning point in my life. As far back as I can remember throughout my adult life I would often feel sad but could never identify why and I could never really cry. I could cry if I watched a Disney® cartoon film but not for any other reason except something significantly upsetting like when I had to take my dog to be put to sleep at the vet.

I realised that before the stroke I was unhappy deep inside. I did a good job of masking that and generally, I had good positive energy (well that's what people said). But, deep down I felt unhappy, and I could never explain why. I would sometimes even have suicidal thoughts but I couldn't ever explain why.

On this particular day when I wrote this post, I played this album for the first time in years and the tears flooded! As the post describes, I felt wave after wave of emotion with each different track. It's an incredible album that flows from one track to another without any breaks. There are no words in the tracks, it is all music only. I would say that it's my favourite album ever. As the music flowed so did my emotions and each track seemed to evoke more tears; more sobbing; but for every track with tears there was a welcome relief; a lessening of the burden that I had been carrying and holding onto like an unwanted cancer; hidden but exceptionally heavy and consuming. The weight was becoming lighter until the tears were tears of joy. I ended up laughing and crying in unison; I was quite a mess I can tell you but the emotional experience was truly awakening. As I listened, I surrendered and released all resistance. God was my co-pilot now. Something has changed inside of me. The internal persistent sadness had gone; the suffering had ceased; I felt lighter and happier. Now the true me could be born again; I had been through a reboot.

Being able to feel and release emotions has been incredible for me as I navigated my recovery. I've always been an emotional person but the ability to feel and release is an entirely new experience for me. I think one of the keys for me is to be able to not attach any meaning to an emotion. This was something that Claire taught me; her emotional intelligence is literally off the charts!

I now acknowledge that if sadness rises in me, then I accept it. I feel the sadness (in this example) and if that results in tears then that's okay, that's probably a good thing because the emotion is moving out of my body. Have you ever heard of the expression that emotion is energy in motion (e-motion)? So feeling and expressing the sadness as tears allows the energy to flow from my body without holding onto and storing that energy. I believe that life-force energy is like water; it wants to flow freely. If it gets blocked, it stagnates, festers and turns bad, creating dis-ease in the body. I often wonder if this could have been part of the cause of my high blood pressure and stroke. I know it's a different way of thinking but I feel that this makes a lot of sense to me. It truly is a holistic way of thinking to complete well-being.

I believe well-being is the continuous flow of life-force divine-intelligent energy (this is God that I refer to a lot). It wants to flow and create; it wants to expand; it is pure unconditional love. Therefore, it follows that well-being in the emotional, physical, mental and spiritual sense is just the start of the picture. Well-being covers everything. Think of the big subjects or topics in your life and add the word well-being at the end and you start to see what I mean; relationship well-being; financial well-being; social well-being. If we analyse the word it makes a lot of sense:

Well-being (or being well) means that we are being well in the sense that "all is well" in our state. It follows then that if all is well that means that everything in our universe is well; it is fully loving and expansive; creative and flowing; this is the ideal state that we can become; just perfect.

Transformation Key: Develop an advanced emotional intelligence

30

19 October 2021: Fatigue

FATIGUE

It really is a thing after a stroke. I never knew how tiring it is for the brain to do simple activities and tasks.

The best way to reduce the fatigue is to move slowly.

My physio has taught me to slow everything down so that I reduce the symptoms of fatigue, dizziness and nausea....and it works

As she keeps telling me, I am my brains teacher, and it likes things to go slowly.

No surprise there then

One of the most challenging movements for me is leaning backwards. If I move at normal speed I feel awful. My physio asked me to rate it out of 5 and it's a maximum of 5/5 for all three symptoms fatigue, dizziness and nausea.

Who would have thought that such a simple thing would be so

> *difficult and cause so much upset in my daily routine?*
> *I guess that's the same for anyone recovering or living with chronic illness. Thank god I'm in the recovering category!!*
> *For now, it's a slow steady progressive recovery... nothing to rush. I have to teach my brain and body slowly.*
> *Slower is Stronger is my new motto and mantra for life.*
> *I think it applies to all aspects of life. in the meantime here's a pic of me trying to smile with straining abs as I slower lower myself without any symptoms*

Brain fatigue is a significant aspect of recovery from any brain injury and stroke is no exception. There's a persistent fogginess and I found that if I had put my brain to work by doing...well anything really... then all I wanted to do having completed the task, was sleep. The fatigue I experienced was unlike anything I'd ever experienced previously. I've been tired before (of course) but this was different; almost indescribable. I'm sure it was the ever-present fog in my thinking that was the primary difference. I suppose the nearest thing to compare would be the tiredness and inability to think following no sleep for days on end. It's the kind of fatigue that quickly induces anxiety and a sense of paranoia; delusions of persecution, jealousy and isolation. In short, it feels horrible.

To ease the burden on the brain I discovered that when I slowed down my activities or tasks I allowed my brain to recover, and the fatigue would not last as long. I figured out that I would rebuild my brain stronger if I slowed things down.

and that it was completely okay to feel exhausted. If I needed to sleep, then that's exactly what I did; I slept. Often I would find I would sleep for hours on end after doing a seemingly trivial set of tasks like getting up, having breakfast, taking my blood pressure, taking my blood pressure medication, having a wash and getting dressed.

The important thing that I understood was that I was in this for the long haul; there was no quick fix. For our modern condition of instant gratification, this long-haul approach can seem counterproductive. We often want the quick pill; the instant remedy; the magic wand to our transformation, healing or recovery. However, rewiring the brain is not a quick fix process, it is based on repetition and consistency, and that meant my brain was going to get very tired. I quickly understood the power of sleep in the healing and transformation process.

When I understood that, I also made sure that I continued to feed my brain with positive affirmations of a strong recovery along with the process of slowing things down and sleeping to ensure the reboot and upgrades I was receiving would be installed correctly and would be 'bug-free'. I didn't want to rewire my brain incorrectly. Have you ever noticed that sometimes after an upgrade of software, certain functions don't work as well as they used to? Well, I guess this is like my upgrade. I didn't want to install functions that didn't work properly any more. What this would mean in real terms was that I had to surrender to the process, accept that I was in for the long haul and I had to give myself grace for the regular periods of sleep.

Transformation Key: Slower + Sleep = Stronger. Transformation will be stronger when you allow yourself to ease into the flow which might mean acceptance of the long road, slowing down tasks and getting plenty of restorative sleep.

31

19 October 2021: I Was Feeling Sad

I was feeling sad

So Claire said "Come on let's get you out "

Yes, my mood immediately lifted.

I put my walking boots on (yes I meant business today)and we set out.

In recent days I'd set some new goals to walk up the track to the woods.

Goal 1: Walk to the tree with the swing and look out across the field towards the western horizon.

Goal 2: Walk to the top of the track (twice as far as goal 1) but return before the wood.

Goal 3: Walk all the way up the track and then around the wood.

> *So this afternoon I did Goal 1!!*
>
> *I'm pleased with this progress. The track is rough and far from level. Today it had the added challenge of long-cut brambles and thorns that made walking a little tricky.*
>
> *But I made it!*
>
> *I used to run this track and wood every morning but this step in my recovery is huge for me mentally...it was just what I needed to lift my mood*

It's a common activity for many people, but goal setting has contributed greatly to my recovery. I've never been one to write down my goals but I'm always setting myself goals in my head. All my goals have been very clear to me and even if my goals have been lofty, I always have a natural ability to break them down into smaller achievable goals. The journey of my recovery has been full of small incremental achievements. When I think of these achievements retrospectively, I realise that these incremental achievements were always in my thoughts and vision. I believe linking thoughts, vision and goals is an important strategy for making significant progress in any endeavour.

In this particular post, I highlighted the goals I'd set with my walking in the local countryside close to my home. I used to run to the woods near our home. I used to run around the woods in all types of weather and unfavourable weather conditions, so the fact that I had yet to even walk to the woods, walking around them seemed like a far-off goal in my mind.

Nevertheless, every endeavour, from walking on the moon to walking to the woods, breaks down into small incremental steps and achievements, and every endeavour starts with a decision and vision of accomplishment.

The mindset has to remain focused on the goal (large or small) to allow the brain to rebuild, regardless of the overall objective. My brain recovery is no different in that respect, I had to start where I was at and I had to take small incremental steps to transform myself into the new version of me that I could envision.

Was it hard?

Yes, it's very hard. Physically, mentally, emotionally, spiritually, financially, and socially; every aspect of life is tested to the maximum extent possible, and then more. It will test you and those who love you, constantly. There will be times when it feels too much. I felt life wasn't fair. Why me? What had I done so wrong that I deserved this?

Goal setting helped overcome those desperate times. Achieving incremental steps always demonstrated to me that I was progressing....and that (above all else) was the objective.

Transformation Key: Having set the vision, break it down into incremental goals and see yourself achieving those goals, and before you know it, your vision starts to become your reality.

32

20 October 2021: A Great Day

A great day

So much to celebrate today:

Connecting with Craig Pankhurst and discovering the incredible work of his charity "A Stroke of Luck". Absolutely genius name with services and work that is invaluable to survivors of stroke. I spent time exploring their website earlier today reading survivor stories - so many young people! Stories that were so relatable to me.

I felt a sense of companionship and understanding. As a stroke survivor himself, reading Craig's own story brought back my own memories that invoked that fear and helplessness from that fateful day.

His work through his charity looks brilliant

I'm so glad to have made this new friend. There will be much more to come from this I'm sure!

Also, following on from yesterday's walking goal achievement, today I set out in a different direction (it was too wet underfoot to attempt the woods today).

I set out towards the farm down the lane.

With Claire accompanying me, we walked to see more of the view to the west and I could really feel the wind on my face.. it felt wonderful. Claire then took me in our VW (soon-to-be camper) to pick up my youngest kids from school.

Physio have said that a ride out like that is good for the brain, although tiring of course.

Once we were home I then walked towards the farm again but with Charlotte this time. It was lovely to hear about school and catch up with her about her life and what's important for her at this time.

I then stayed for dinner with the family which was amazing. Good ol' sausages, mash, broccoli and gravy. Always a winner!!

Thank you Claire xx

All in all, a great day

I remember this day like it was yesterday. It's funny how certain memories are etched into the mind more than others. I think it was the fact that I got to spend a bit of one-on-one time catching up with Charlotte. It was a difficult time for all the kids but I think Charlotte felt it more acutely.

As a 15 year girl the mental anguish upon her was severe

and Claire poured love into Charlotte to allow Charlotte the space to fully express herself. I cannot thank Claire enough for that ongoing outpouring of love towards Charlotte in that period. I was not in any state to mentally or emotionally cope with the needs of my children as I was too wrapped up in my recovery. Understandably, Charlotte ended up hating the stroke during this period, and I can see why. She was going through her challenges in life, and then there was her dad in a difficult condition himself, unable to be any support like I thought a father should be. Poor girl. If I could get that time back to make amends then I would. But we're all here to learn some big lessons. Luckily, with Claire's help, Charlotte navigated her way through the difficult times to find her former 'bubbly' self. She's an incredible young lady who has built massive resilience, stands up for what she believes in and doesn't take any crap off anyone; I'm so proud of her. She will have learnt so many lessons from that period and as hard as it feels at the time, all the lessons are for us (at some level) and her soul will have benefitted for this life or others to come.

This was also the day that I connected with Craig Pankhurst, CEO of A Stroke Of Luck, also known as ASL. Craig started the charity ASL as a result of experiencing stroke himself and like me, his attitude was centred on stroke survival rather than being a victim of stroke. This perspective is so important; survival not victim!! Craig wanted to help other survivors of stroke by helping them connect with personal trainers who specialise in rehabilitation for Stroke survivors. This is brilliant work. My recovery has incorporated exercise throughout. Exercise is not only good for physical well-being and brain recovery but it is also vital for mental and emotional well-being.

On the ASL website, there are numerous stories from other Stroke survivors and I recall spending an entire afternoon reading through the other stroke survivor stories on the ASL website. One thing that struck me was how young so many of the people were who had submitted their own stories. People in their 20's, 30's and 40's as well as others like me at 50 and beyond. Whilst so many of the stories were distressing, they all carried a sense of hope for recovery and rehabilitation. For me, the target was more than recovery and rehabilitation; this was an opportunity to transform entirely. I had no idea what that transformation might end up looking like; although plenty of thoughts have since come to mind, like my approach to goal setting, I have a vision but I am accepting that the flow of life will allow that vision to unfold as I progress towards it. Most of all (and it's a cliche) the experience is in the journey towards the vision and destination, and not necessarily the destination itself.

Transformation Key: The richness of the experience is in the journey and not the destination.

33

22 October 2021:
Reflecting

Reflecting

It's been a quiet end to the week. I don't do quiet very well, I tend to like achieving things and feeling a sense of accomplishment, but quiet is all ok too.

The quietness gives me time to reflect on a number of things:

how lucky I am to be surrounded by so much love and support from my A-team led by my rock and love Claire. She knows exactly how I'm feeling, when to push me and when to back off, what I need, when I need it, she just knows without me having to say a word... I would be totally lost without Claire and her unwavering love and support. I will pay you back in bucketloads when I am able baby I promise.

The kindness of Claire's mum and dad, Anita and Roger, who have generously given up their home to allow me to recover in peace whilst still being in the home environment. Thank you both for your continued kindness.

The love and support from friends and family who have cooked and transported for our family - meals, and hospital visits during my first two weeks post-stroke. So grateful for your help and lovely meals too.

For all the messages and comments of support, prayers and love on social media and in my inbox. These really are treasured. I've loved reading them all. For the financial generosity of my immediate CFX family who raised funds in BTC (Bitcoin) for our family to help us during this period. Both Claire and I are self-employed and have no backup plan to bail us out when I am not able to work. We are totally reliant on her income!

For the new introductions, friends and connections I've made across the week that have provided me with a glimpse of potentially new avenues to allow me to give back (when I am able). Helping out with supporting other survivors of stroke. Raising awareness. Fundraising. Speaking. Writing. Whatever form that takes, who knows?

Additionally, having a quiet day has allowed me to read (I love to read). My brother, Phil, told me about the book, "Captain Tom's Life Lessons"

Today I finished it. A wonderful read and such wisdom from this great and humble man. What a perfect way to round off the week. Reading such wisdom from a man whose life spanned over 100 years and whose commitment raised over £1M for the

NHS during the height of the UK Covid lockdowns.
I cannot recommend this little book enough.
Love to all!

It was becoming more obvious to me that my sense of gratitude for other people's generosity was being heightened all the time. This recovery was going to take a while and I had to learn to surrender to the time it would take. That didn't mean I simply consented to this "fate", but I felt it pointless to try to push my way through the recovery. I had no previous experience of brain injury recovery to call upon so I decided that I would recover when my body wanted me to recover and that also meant that I had to surrender to the process of recovery, however long that would take. That was a hard thing for me to come to terms with but put bluntly, I had no choice, I had to get used to it. So in that sense, surrender was the only option.

Alongside that sense of surrender, was the overwhelming sense of gratitude that was starting to build inside of me. Gratitude for so much; the love and generosity of family and friends; the words of encouragement and support from social media friends and connections; the meals for the family delivered by friends; the donations of bitcoin made by other members of our network marketing team; but most of all the gratitude for being alive; yes, life was difficult at this moment, but I was alive! That is what mattered the most.

Surrender and gratitude are huge steps in my recovery journey.

The opposite of surrender is to keep pushing through, which could be an approach that I probably used to favour but brain recovery requires a softer approach. Softer in the sense of forgiveness and patience. It would be easy to give up so that meant I also had to have a sense of determination, but it was balanced. Determination balanced with Surrender. It's an odd mix, but it's the only mix that gave me any chance of recovery.

Transformation Key: Learn to balance determination with surrender to remove internal resistance to transformation.

Home - Family Home

34

24 October 2021: Massive Progress

Massive progress

So yesterday I achieved some amazing goals and progress.

1. *Claire suggested that I come over to join her and the kids for dinner and then to sleep over together (Claire and I, not the kids) We did it, and all that I was concerned about was taken away.*
2. *One of the goals that I'd set when I first went into hospital was to be able to throw the rugby ball with the kids like I used to do.*

So it wasn't quite to the same level but yesterday, I spent time with the kids in the garden passing and throwing the rugby ball to one another.

Today, we've made the decision to move me permanently back into the family home. I am so grateful to have had the use of Roger and Anita's wonderful annex with everything on one level; the peace and quiet; the sanctuary in which to build strength and confidence in my physical, mental and emotional abilities.

But the time has come to become fully integrated back with the family into the family home, with kids, dog, stairs and other minute details that I had previously feared.

Today, I'm truly home.

Claire is an absolute champion and I cannot thank her or praise her enough. I feel so much love from her and I to her

Throughout my recovery, she has been there to make everything happen. Today was no different. She rallied the help of the girls and moved me back into the family home.

Done just like that. Thanks, girls

So now I have the noise and bustle of family life, I can share the living room with Toby (the dog)....let the next stage of recovery commence!!!

It feels amazing to be fully home!

So this was the day I came back to the family home; the day I was fully reintegrated back into family life. I was fearful at the thought of being around the hustle and bustle of family life. I had been in a quiet place to allow my recovery to form a foundation and I wasn't entirely sure if I was ready to make the next move to be around people, although in this case, it was family and loved ones. Nevertheless, I was nervous. An injured and recovering brain can play all sorts of anxiety tricks and I was feeling that anxiety.

This is where my gratitude for Claire and her ability to push me when she knew I was ready. Claire is not medically qualified but she trusts her intuition and she knew I was ready. She knew that I would cope ok and she was running the show and organising the help of our kids.

I remember the relief of being truly home; my initial recovery on my own in the annexe had been great but now I was ready to commence the next stage; integration. The thought of taking the next steps and integrating helped me overcome any anxious feelings. My determination coupled with Claire's intuitive 'push' helped make the transition to home life a success.

On that same day, I also started to throw the rugby ball with the kids. Before the stroke, I would throw and kick the rugby ball for my son William, and Eva and Logan would sometimes join in. I missed throwing the ball with William so much; it's a great bonding experience for a father and son (and in this case my future step-children as well).

When I was in Swindon GWH and working with the physio team, I said that one of my goals was to throw and kick the rugby ball with William again; I was determined to achieve that goal.

This day was the first day when I did that again. William was amazing with me. He could see that I was in such a frail state so he took it easy with me by gently throwing the ball to me and we passed it around the circle of Logan, Eva, William and me. In comparison to our pre-stroke kicks and throws it was like taking baby steps all over again but it was a start; the full ability would return one day. It would only take a moment; and that moment might take days, weeks, months or years. I had no idea, but we had started and that was the main thing.

Transformation Key: Step out of your comfort zone. Your comfort zone will only keep you trapped where you are.

35

28 October 2021: Walked
The Dog

Walked the dog !!!

Celebrating another milestone this afternoon!!

Claire was busy (as usual), I was not (recovery underway) so I said, "I'll think I'll walk the dog."

Claire: Shall I come with you, just to the stile, shall I get one of the neighbours to keep an eye out for you???

Me: Nope I'll be fine thanks

Claire: Do you want to do it or would you prefer not to do it?

Me: I want to babe - well my head is saying yes even though my stomach is churning and I feel sick

Claire: Fear?

Me: No idea! Don't think so.

So off I went, just me and Toby (the dog).

He was brilliant. He didn't pull on the lead at all. I think he knew he would have pulled me over if he had! So he was super gentle with me and I got to take him across the field in front of our house (we're so lucky to have this countryside on our doorstep).

We didn't walk too far but far enough that we both enjoyed it and felt better for doing it

Happy days

Walking Toby, our dog has been amazing therapy and helped my recovery. This was the day that I took my first walk alone with Toby. As with any first, the initial thought of doing so was worse than the actual act.

I recall those tentative steps with Toby at my side. He walked gently with me as if he knew I was frail and could easily lose my balance.

I always took my phone with me for several reasons. I suppose the obvious reason was in case I fell and needed to call Claire. Luckily that never happened. The other reason is my love of music, and specifically, as I walk in the fields, I love peaceful meditation music. At the time of writing this, my go-to playlist is called Musical Therapy. I push the phone into the top pocket of my coat and play the playlist as I walk. The combination of peaceful therapeutic music combined with the sounds of nature creates a state of bliss in my mind. I've met neighbours whilst out walking and as I stop the chat, there is beautiful blissful music playing in the air as if my magic. I can imagine the thoughts of these neighbours as I bid them goodbye after chatting. They might think, "Wow, where did that beautiful music come from? It was like a moment of heaven." "Indeed, it certainly was heaven, and you're welcome", I would think and chuckle to myself.

Walking out alone with Toby dog was a major milestone. It gave me a sense of independence; it helped me create greater stability in my walking; it gave me direct access to fresh air; it improved my mental health; the benefits are countless and tremendous. Even if walking is difficult, I would recommend getting outside whenever and however that is possible. I feel desperately sorry for those without access to nature or the ability to get outside in the fresh air. During the pandemic and the lockdowns I was so grateful to live in a place with such immediate access to nature; it is an absolute blessing!

Transformation Key: Get outside and walk in nature if possible. Consider playing your favourite playlist for accompaniment.

36

29 October 2021: Goal 3 Smashed

Goal 3 smashed.

To say I'm pleased is an understatement!!

Last week I walked up towards the woods as far as the tree and back. I posted how that was goal 1 of 3.

Well, I've just returned from another walk with the dog but this time I walked around the wood.

I couldn't have picked a more traitorous time of the year.

As autumn (fall) is upon us and it poured with rain about 2 hours before my walk, the ground in the woods is slippery with muddy puddles, wet branches, and soggy leaves covering any sign of a path. Perhaps a covering of snow would have been worse!

It was challenging.

I'm sure my physio-therapy team would have been impressed had they seen the obstacles in my way.

I didn't go fast (I can't) but I slowly made my way around the slippery woodland path...it was physiotherapy out in nature (the best version).

So I have to say I'm chuffed to bits (happy) and proud of my progress. I can really start to imagine other goals being achieved very quickly.

There's absolutely no doubt in my mind that taking an approach of slower but stronger combined with self-care (i.e. sleep when I need to) combined with a bit of courage to walk with fears, has all worked to accelerate my recovery. Recovery is far from complete (no way!) but this week has seen huge steps forward

My family and I are blessed to live close to a beautiful area of woodland. It is not managed and therefore it manages itself. Every time I visit to walk around it's different; it is a place of continuous change in a natural setting. There is so much to see, but the obvious points of a year in the woods are punctuated by the seasons.

Spring is my favourite time of the year no matter where I am, but this is a magic time in the woods because I can witness the new spring flowers pushing their way through the woodland floor to mark the arrival of warmer days with a small pin-prick of colour that then spreads to create a stunning impact. It is also a time to witness the new growth of leaves and buds on the branches of the trees. I love finding new growth as there's a visceral sense of achievement from the new growth.; achievement for surviving and growing through the cold winter months and then making the appearance in spring. As the year progresses, the change of temperature is marked within the woods by the woodland life.

In the Autumn and Winter large branches and even whole trees will break and fall. Luckily, I have not been in the woods at the time of a tree falling or a large branch coming down, but the effect on the route around the wood can be significant. Overnight, a former path trodden for years will disappear beneath a large tree or branch. Once that happens the inhabitants of the wood (including walkers like me) have no choice but to create new paths in the undergrowth.

It's the same for the plants in the woods. When a tree has fallen, the plants will always find a way to find the sunlight and grow; it's the natural order of repair and recovery.

Amid springtime in April, the floor of the entire woods becomes an abundant display of stunning bluebells. It is a jaw-dropping sight that takes the breath away. The abundance is short-lived and lasts for about 4 weeks starting in late March to continue through April. The woodland floor looks like a purple magical fairyland with the trodden path showing a prominent brown almost lighting the way through the magical purple haze of bluebells.

The woods have provided me with a sense of reflection and a great metaphor for my recovery; no matter the circumstances, there is a way to reach the light and recover, in whatever form that looks like.

Transformation Key: Observe the wonder of nature wherever you can. It reflects the pure natural state of continuous growth and recovery throughout the seasons.

37

1 November 2021: Goals

GOALS

Another goal that Claire and I set while I was in hospital was that I would be walking along THE RIDGEWAY as soon as I could.

When I look back at my first steps in hospital I find it amazing that I am now walking "the ridge" and embracing the weather!

Yes, this goal was shattered over the weekend just gone. Whilst today, I am really tired and feeling a bit glum, when I consider that Saturday afternoon walk, I am really pleased and feel blessed.

Later, I will walk out with Toby (our dog) which will lift my mood. Exercise is a great enhancer of mood..and getting out in nature does the same.

As I write this post, I'm listening to some great new Anjunadeep

releases, which are lifting my mood even further.
Some great mood-lifting lessons here:

Accomplishment of Goals - Set those goals and push through slowly but with strength and determination.

Consistency with positive habits - take a walk, get outside in nature.

Do more of what feels good - listening to music can be so uplifting.

I cannot emphasise this enough, but walking out in the fresh air is amazing! If physically walking is difficult then try to seek assistance to enable you to get outside as often as possible. The fresh air is the best medicine there is, and getting outside is by far the best physiotherapy you can do if you are recovering from a stroke.

I have to caveat that statement with the understanding that everyone who has survived and is recovering from a stroke will have a unique experience. For the haemorrhage within the cerebellum of my brain which caused me an intense loss of balance, walking was unbelievably difficult in the early days of recovery. Venturing outside, despite the weather conditions, was very important for my recovery journey. If you can manage walking (even slightly) then push yourself to walk outside as often as you can. It is very common to have people left with more severe and permanent disabilities but this does not mean that getting outside is precluded from your life experience. It will be difficult. It was difficult for me, I couldn't walk at all in the hospital I was bedridden for over a week and had to learn how to walk again, but you can do anything if you want to.

As I write this it is now over 7 months since the stroke and I walk twice a day even on the days I work at the computer. I find that if I don't walk, my sense of imbalance gets worse, whereas walking (especially across the fields or in the woods) helps.

Transformation Key: If you are able, walk outside as often as possible, ideally at least twice a day if you can.

38

2 November 2021: "Have You Brought Your Coat?"

> *"Have you brought your coat?"*
> were the words I used to greet my Physio Therapist, Sue, this morning.
> As I've stated many times in my posts, the best therapy for my recovery from stroke has been to have a good walk out in the fresh air and countryside...it cannot be beaten.
> So today, I took my physiotherapist for a local walk.
> She was impressed and re-affirmed the progression I had made in the 7 weeks since S-Day (as I've now decided to call it).
> When I think back to S-Day and the immediate chaos that ensued, I am amazed at the difference.
> I couldn't walk, talk or sit up in bed. Jeez, I nearly died, had it not been for the miracle that kept me alive. I had probes in my

arteries and into my brain

My life was in the hands of God and the incredibly talented team operating the CT probe and associated equipment. I had no idea at the time just how close to the end I was.

Now, 7 weeks later, I'm asking my physiotherapist to accompany me on a walk in the countryside!!! Waaahh amazing progress

As we walked I noticed some Apples outside a neighbouring cottage. Put outside by the owner as a "Freebie" to any budding cooks that happen to walk past.

I grabbed a few and said to Sue, "I'm going to make a crumble, can you help me take a couple, please?"...and so I did, well I actually made two crumbles in fact

Darn tasty too with a scoop of ice cream

As I gained more strength and rediscovered the enjoyment of the act of being in the fresh air and walking, I switched up my physiotherapy sessions with my team.

They all soon got into the habit of bringing their coats and wellies to accompany me on my walks. I still did the physiotherapy they had planned for me but my preference was always to walk, so I made it become part of my physiotherapy recovery plan.

I think the message to take from this is to never be afraid to take control of your destiny and work with those who are assigned to help you. Don't sit back passively and wait for everything to come to you, the secret is to take some action and take the initiative.

I'm pretty sure that my physio-therapy team didn't have many people like me who insisted on going for a walk together.

Also, never be afraid to introduce something interesting or something that makes the event a little different. As I'm fortunate to live in the English countryside, Apples and Pears are in good supply in the Autumn months. On this particular occasion, I walked past a neighbour's house and saw some Apples in a wheelbarrow to take free of charge. This then led to the opportunity to cook a couple of Apple crumbles. I'm certain that walking, collecting apples and then cooking the crumbles all helped with my brain recovery in some way, maybe a small way or perhaps it was far more significant, but it was all a sign of progress, and that in itself builds more recovery. The crumbles were lovely too with a tasty dollop of ice cream!

Transformation Key: Take control of your destiny and never be afraid of mixing up the set plan. You are always in control!

39

6 November 2021: 2 Months Ago Today

> *2 months ago today*
>
> *I had a bleed into my brain, the stroke hit me out of nowhere!!*
> *Bamm*
>
> *One moment I was fine, the next my life had changed instantly.*
> *Exactly 2 months ago to the day/moment, I was unable to stand,*
> *I couldn't see or focus on anything, I was violently sick, I fell*
> *into unconsciousness, everything changed....*
>
> *But not forever!!!*
>
> *Here I am 2 months later, and I am now living with a perma-*
> *nent sense of imbalance but....I am alive!! I survived!!*
>
> *Yes, life is radically different, I have to accept that and some-*
> *times that is hard to accept, why me?! what the F did I do to*
> *deserve this ?!*

I can't lie, sometimes these thoughts do run through my mind, I can feel pretty glum sometimes but the thing that keeps me going and picks me up is remembering that I survived!! And I am recovering

Will I return to life as it was? God knows, truly only God knows, I certainly don't but I am grateful for every precious moment that is presented to me. I love walking outdoors, I have a renewed sense of learning (I've always loved learning but this has deepened in the last few weeks), and I have a new sense of not giving a toss what anybody thinks of me... (I'm done with all that crap...life is literally too short!)

So here's to life !! With all its madness and uncertainty. I embrace every moment and I am grateful for everything..I take nothing for granted.

With love

If you're reading this as a Stroke Survivor, there will be moments when you will want to give up. There will be moments when you'll feel anger and a sense of 'why me?' This is completely normal. You will inevitably feel grief for the loss of your former self. This is also completely normal. There are multiple stages in the grieving process and the process of recovery and rebuilding one's brain is also accompanied by the process of grieving. You'll go through an emotional shitstorm, but I found that the solid foundation of remembering and being so profoundly grateful that I was alive, helped to keep me focused on recovery during those very dark times.

This is, once again, why it's so important to get outside in nature as much as you can because it will help your mental and emotional well-being. I find that being in nature every day provides a daily dose of vitamin D and a gorgeous source of energy.

It was during the darker days that I would turn to my inner voice of compassion, grace and forgiveness to help reassure me that despite the length of the recovery journey, I knew in my heart that I would ultimately recover and reboot, but thereafter the journey of transformation would never stop. Continuous change is inevitable. The cells of our body are regenerating and transforming at every moment, so change is a constant occurrence. With that knowing in my heart, I was mentally refuelled to keep going, and gently but firmly, pushed on with my recovery.

Transformation Key: Try not to focus on the loss of your former self, but rather, switch your focus on the possibilities and potentialities held within the transformation.

40

7 November 2021:
Cooking

Cooking

Today I've taken on the task of cooking the Sunday dinner for the family.

It's tiring but I love preparing and cooking food for others...and after the stroke, it gives me a great sense of accomplishment.

So on the menu today we have slow-cooked braising beef with mash and something (haven't decided yet - either peas, green beans or broccoli, or maybe all three) and sausages, mash and peas for the kids (who don't like the braised beef).

All the prep is done and I'm now taking 20 minutes to chill out and catch up on the rugby (Autumn Nations Series - yes)

In the few years before the stroke, I had always enjoyed

cooking for the family. That was not always the case mind you. Before I met Claire, I would have said that I wasn't particularly keen on cooking. It wasn't that I couldn't cook; I could, but I wasn't that interested in being creative in the kitchen.

As my recovery grew from strength to strength, I started to enjoy some of the tasks that my former self could have enjoyed, such as cooking.

Considering that my balance was still not 100% stable, I did laugh at myself for handling all the kitchen knives without cutting myself, although it did take quite a lot of concentration to peel and slice the vegetables successfully!

Doing the cooking for the family did give me a sense of accomplishment although it was tiring and I recall that on one or two occasions I did completely mess up the timing. I soon discovered that trying to multi-task had become a very difficult thing for me to do, especially if something unexpected occurred. I figured out various strategies to support my recovering brain so that I wouldn't get too stressed out by my confusion from multitasking. Simple things would help, like using timers and making notes, for example.

Transformation Key: Use tools to help you carry out multiple tasks at once so that you give your transforming brain a fighting chance. It also reduces any additional pressure and stress.

41

7 November 2021: A great walk but I was physically exhausted

A great walk but I was physically exhausted

Although it was only a stroll this walk pushed me!!

When I got home I had to sleep

On the one hand, I was pleased as punch (8 weeks ago I was nearly dead and now I'm walking these walks - amazing recovery) but on the other hand I feel down (because 9 weeks ago doing this would have been super easy).

I can't help but compare before stroke with after stroke! I don't want to and it's not mentally healthy to do so, but I can't help it.

> *Maybe tomorrow I'll see the positive side again and see the progress*

There will be a great temptation to compare your old/former self with the version that you are during recovery but try not to compare and judge yourself as it can be quite damaging.

There is an acceptance that must take place. Yes, life is very different, and you can be pissed off and angry if you want to, but please do not hold onto this angry emotion, just let it go! I know that is way easier to say than do; believe me, I know! When you accept what is rather than what you think it should be, and when you give up holding onto some form of damaging self-judgement, then the true recovery and transformation has a chance to start in earnest.

At the end of the day, continuously thinking and comparing yourself pre-stroke vs. post-stroke could emotionally mess with your head, so don't do it, or else you could seriously jeopardise your recovery.

If you do find yourself comparing and feeling angry about the loss of your former self, then breathe deeply, scream and shout at the wind, cry, and just do whatever it takes to let go of the emotion without hurting anyone else, because if you don't then that emotion could hurt you. Transformation can only start when you let go of the ego-self that wants to protect you. However in that protection, the ego-self of doubt, fear, judgement and comparison will hold you back from a transformation that is beautiful, truly profound and life-changing. There is probably something profoundly beautiful on the other side of the fear, doubt and comparison. It might look crazy stupid to your (so-called) rational mind but become willing to embrace the new version of you. The less mental resistance there is the greater the potential.

Transformation Key: Give up all fear-based comparisons of your former self with your current transforming self. The comparison could cause you to hold an unhealthy self-image and self-judgement of your transforming self.

42

8 November 2021: "Alexa, play Rush, Manhattan Project"

"Alexa, play Rush, Manhattan Project"

I sat alone on the kitchen stool having my breakfast and then I wanted to listen to music that I listened to as a teenager.
And I wanted it really loud.
Claire was out and she returned to find me with tears pouring down my face as I was completely lost in the music...I've always found music so emotive
I had been transported back 40 years to a moment when my mum had found me lying on the lounge floor with my head between the stereo speakers playing the same track, again, very

loud. I recall she turned around and walked out, shrugging her shoulders as if to say "Oh well, never mind" lol

It felt amazing to let the tears flow again this morning. There was no real meaning to the tears

neither happy nor sad, they were just tears, which was great I had been transported back to a time with no stress, no history. There was no meaning, no attachment, these were just tears carrying away something that needed to shift I guess. All good, all fine, it just was and nothing more...and it felt fantastic! Thank you, Rush.

And now to get on with the rest of the day...what a perfect start Have a great day

Releasing emotions is a wonderful tool for mastery of self-development and self-actualisation. We hold onto past emotions associated with old wounding (hurt) and very often, we will protect ourselves from further hurt by not allowing that emotion to flow through and out. We develop strategies to avoid the pain and hurt rather than simply letting the emotion flow through and out of the body. Holding onto the emotions and burying them through avoidance can cause a lot of damage. It is so very common to find that therapists advise the opposite and I suppose in certain circumstances the opposite approach might be true. But I had experienced serious brain trauma and no one except Claire was there to help me. Thank God for Claire I say for without her skill and guidance it might have all been a very different story.

I believe that everything in the universe is energy and in that same way, I consider emotions held in the body as energy that is stuck. Furthermore, I believe that stuck energy is not healthy and will result in dis-ease in the body.

I don't advocate a full reenactment or recollection of the situation that caused the hurt but I do advocate releasing the emotion. Several techniques help such as EFT (Emotional Freedom Technique) otherwise known as Tapping, can help. I find that EFT works on one occasion but not on others and I am yet to determine a pattern to identify when it will be effective for me and when it won't.

Another approach that Claire has taught me is to allow myself to feel the emotion but then not attach any meaning to the emotion. I have found this approach to be very effective. Additionally, if the emotion is frustration then I find that having a good rant about it can work. I don't mean moaning in some gossip kind of way (that is unhealthy). I find that just 5 or 10 minutes of ranting can release the frustration and it is replaced by a lighter feeling in the body. Claire is superb at being on the receiving end of a good rant as she is emotionally wise enough to know that my ranting is not directed at her even though I might be ranting at her. If you don't have an emotionally wise partner like I have in Claire, then I would recommend getting a cat to rant at. The point of ranting for me is not to amplify the negative emotion but eradicate it and allow the void that is created to be replaced by a lightness, aka love.

As a concept, just feeling the emotion without attaching meaning is relatively easy to grasp but then actually not attaching meaning to an emotion that needs to flow can be quite difficult at first, but I've found that taking deep breaths and blowing out whilst the emotion moves helps clear it from the body. This might sound crazy to some people but to those people, I would recommend having an open mind to the possibility that this might work and to remove any preconceived resistance to this approach.

I have advised many other Stroke survivors with this technique to release emotions that are stuck in the body, and they've all been very grateful for the help. I haven't been able to form any conclusive evidence through scientific study but there is plenty of anecdotal evidence to support the effectiveness of this technique.

Transformation Key: Allow old emotions to pass through the body without attaching any meaning or judgment. Holding on to past trauma and associated emotions can lead to dis-ease.

43

⊱❦⊰

11 November 2021: Following My Soul Takes Courage

Following my soul... takes courage!

My ability to "work" has been seriously impaired since I survived the stroke.

Quite simply I get exhausted by almost anything challenging. The physical and mental impact is unbelievable.

Yesterday, a Director of Talent from a successful SaaS software company reached out (on LinkedIN) asking to speak about helping them with a role to help them build out/shape and lead a Value Engineering capability

What a perfect role for me! I've been banging on about Business Value for years, built models and training programs, ran workshops for large corporates etc, so perfect except timing...I am in no state to undertake such a commitment and the thought of selling myself and enslaving myself for hours everyday makes me freak out and want to vomit

God gave me this stroke to make me stop.

I had been slowly killing myself throughout my entire career trying to prove something to someone...I mean WTF! There comes a point when we have to listen to the guidance and this is exactly that time. I'm taking time to recover slowly with strength. I mean Jeez I have no choice, I'm constantly in a state of imbalance, I can't do much of anything that I used to do these days, and I have to accept that with grace and humility.

So somewhat regretfully, I had to gracefully turn down the offer to speak about building a brand new Value Engineering capacity, I have to focus on myself first, even if that means not earning a steady income and all the uncertainty that can bring....I have to follow my soul.

This morning having finished my physio workout, (and slept) I am completing my first exercise in my drawing training course.

I have no idea if it will lead to any success but I have to follow my soul and fulfil my desire to draw.

Drawing seems a lot less taxing on me than anything else at the moment...and I have a goal to draw all the illustrations for my children's book series, "The Adventures of Toby and Bentley". More on this goal to come (stay tuned...)

The kind Talent Director understood the timing challenge and said that the door was always open in the future so who knows, but for now, I'll put pencil to paper and get creative.

Several years before the stroke, I had built a successful career in the Technology SaaS (software as a service) industry. In the first two decades of this century, I had been a co-founder and held senior positions in several software companies. I had been Director of Customer Services and Vice President of Global Customer Experience at the heights of that career in 2010 and 2014. I started my own consultancy business in 2019 and navigated the global Coronavirus Pandemic of 2020 with new contracts about to start again in September 2021, and then boom, stroke! So here I was now in late 2021 wondering what the heck I was going to do? If I had been stressed out before, I was now feeling the full force of stress again. I had no idea what I was going to do; I had no idea how we were going to pay our household bills; it was a very worrying time. I had always been the typical provider of the household. I was proud of my accomplishments but where had it all got me? Of course, there were many lessons and vast wisdom but in terms of life and what matters, I would say, the answer to that soul-searching question was...erm, nowhere actually! That's the stark truth and perhaps I had manifested this stroke as a means of stopping that treadmill. I could have thought of slightly less impactful ways but hey sometimes the universe responds in very mysterious ways that might appear to make no sense at first.

Whilst it was very worrying, it was also a period when I had to completely surrender to the situation. I had no option but to focus 100% on my recovery. I found myself handing everything over to a higher power and letting go of the worry. In the process of letting go, I found myself drawn into new interests or interests that I had suppressed for years. I turned to drawing and I started an online training course teaching me the skills to draw.

I pursued it for a while and I enjoyed it I know that one day I will pick it up again and complete the training course. I'm interested in many things and it is not unusual for me to be learning multiple things simultaneously. At that particular time during my recovery, I didn't have the energy to pursue or learn multiple things at once, so it had to be just drawing for the moment, and after each lesson, I would sleep. My brain found the learning exhausting.

Transformation Key: Allow yourself to explore new interests without any judgment if you wish to move on and explore something else. Life is all about experiences and exploring what we want to pursue.

44

12 November 2021: Blood Pressure

Blood Pressure

Every morning between 7:30 and 9:30 am Monitoring my BP has become an essential part of my morning routine.

I recall one of the doctors in the hospital saying that my target reading should be 130/80.

It's not quite there yet, but with meds combined with my mindfulness practice and focus on a good diet, I know it will get there.

The doctors and consultants in the hospital said they could find no other cause for my stroke other than the ridiculously high blood pressure. It shot up to 200+ / 150+ when I had the stroke - crazy high!!!!

Sometimes we have to introduce or adopt new habits into our routines - and it might be a matter of life or death. Whether we like the new habits or not, we must do them! Better that than the alternative right?

The image of the monitor shows my BP reading this morning - yay, close to my target

I also added a bowl of porridge with blueberries into the mix for a super healthy breakfast. Porridge oats are brilliant for reducing blood pressure and blueberries are great for the brain - having both for breakfast seems like a good idea to me - and it's tasty too

So let's hear it for good habits !!!

"Go good habits!!"

The brain haemorrhage that I experienced was said to be caused by excessively high blood pressure or medically called hypertension. The trouble with hypertension is that it doesn't often show any signs. This was the case with me. However in April 2017 (4.5 years before the stroke) I spent 24 hours in hospital having had severe chest pains and high blood pressure.

I was medicated at the time and I took many other precautionary measures including a good diet etc. In short, I led a fairly modest and healthy lifestyle. I didn't smoke, I didn't drink alcohol excessively, I moderated and watched my salt intake and I kept myself fit at the gym but I did find myself suffering from stress and anxiety from all manner of things. After 3 months of medication combined with 6 months of mindfulness practice (so by the end of 2017), I had managed to keep my blood pressure down under 130/80. I spoke to my doctor and I decided that I could drop the medication. At that time, I didn't want to be medicated for the rest of my life. However, what I failed to do was periodically monitor my blood pressure from that point moving forward... oh boy, big mistake!

I had gone through a distressful divorce in 2015, I had started my own business in 2019 (just before the global pandemic), and I was constantly worried about money, paying the bills and trying to provide for the family. Looking back on it now, I carried a lot of stress in my mind and body; I constantly questioned my self-worth and I felt I had to make everything perfect for everyone, all of which is completely self-defeating and ultimately self-destructive. I failed to monitor my blood pressure properly, so I guess the hypertension crept up on me and crept up higher and higher until bang!

As a result of the stroke, I had no choice but to accept the medication that was prescribed to me and get into the habit of periodically checking my blood pressure.

I've changed medication several times in the months following the stroke. At first, the medication read like a grocery list of items but upon leaving the hospital I stabilised onto a prescription of drugs that I had to take morning and night. After several months I realised that the drugs were having side effects that included ankle swelling and water retention in the body. I also questioned whether there was an erectile dysfunction issue as well. After visiting my doctor and talking through the issues I was prescribed an alternative to one of the drugs. It seemed to have a positive effect on the side effects, whilst still working to maintain a stabilised and lowering blood pressure.

When taking my blood pressure I have now noted several important factors:

I take at least three readings. Invariably the first reading will be a little higher than the second and third.

I breathe intentionally as I take the reading. This typically will see an improvement in the result. I breathe in through the nose, hold for 3 seconds and then breathe out through the mouth. I find this helps calm my nervous system and allows me to gain greater control of my body. I do this type of breathing at points throughout my day as well; again, all to calm my nervous system and keep my blood pressure in a stabilised safe state.

I ensure the monitor is positioned at the same height (or thereabouts) as my heart.

I try to take my blood pressure at a consistent time of the day. For me, this is just after rising from bed and washing in the morning but before my morning yoga, pilates, strength training and before the morning medication.

I record my blood pressure readings in a blood pressure/ health App. It doesn't do anything fancy but it allows me to quickly observe 7-day and 30-day averages at a glance.

I have noticed that if I take the reading after my morning workout routine (yoga, pilates, strength training with associated breathing work) then the reading will be slightly lower.

At the point of writing this, it is over 1 year since the stroke and I still monitor my blood pressure every day using the approach listed above. Today (October 13, 2022) my reading was 110/75. Yes, completely and unequivocally in the Normal zone. I have tracked my blood pressure every single day for the best part of the year and not only recorded the results on the App on my phone but also on a spreadsheet so that I could produce graphs, charts and monthly trends over the year. The results are shown at the back of the book.

Transformation Key: Transformation might require following new routines. Don't be dismissive of new transformative habits.

45

13 November 2021: 9
Weeks Ago To The Day

9 weeks ago to the day I was dying!!!

It was sheer hell, knowing I was seriously f..ked, but unable to communicate at all. The rugby posts (normally vertically upright) were spinning around, I had to shut my eyes and couldn't open them again for 4 days. Nothing made any sense! The family event at the local rugby club has turned into a day from hell for me.

Urgh... even thinking about it now makes me feel sick and shiver with fear.

Today, Claire and I spent the afternoon in our local park enjoying the gorgeous colours of the autumn trees.

Stunning.

I had an overarching sense of appreciation for my life, for the

> *beauty of nature and for the incredible recovery journey that I*
> *am on accompanied by the most supportive, loving woman in*
> *the world.*
> *On some days, this journey is hard, but on days like today, it's*
> *completely beautiful*

When I look back at posts like this one, I remember so many aspects of my journey, from the brain haemorrhage itself to the journey during recovery. Throughout the process of recovery, especially since being able to get outside, I have had a profound appreciation for nature.

I've always been a lover of nature. I grew up in the countryside. I was a lad who played with my friends in the fields. We made dens, climbed trees, sledging in the snow, stacked bales of straw in the summer and had mud bomb fights amongst those very same stacked bales. Country life and the countryside is in my DNA.

Nature always demonstrates the perfect cycle of renewal and even in death, the beauty of nature is pure brilliance.

We witness the autumnal colours before winter takes hold with its cold winds and lower temperatures. I used to feel melancholy when the autumn and winter months arrived; I'd feel a sense of loss but in recent years I've seen the beauty in the autumn and winter months. The fading light would disrupt my natural tendency to feel vibrant and alive. I recall a few years ago I used to use a SAD (seasonal affective disorder) lamp during the months with fading light to help restore my mood. In the autumn and winter of 2021/22, I had every reason to feel down, but I resisted the urge to feel low, I had more pressing things to focus on; my recovery with the love of my life by my side.

It was easy to let circumstances get me down. It was under-standable to feel low sometimes, and that was ok. When those moments arose I just forgave myself and tried to see the beauty in what could otherwise look quite depressing. For example, I used to see the autumn leaves dying and rotting, whereas now I see the beauty in either their radiant colours or the beauty in what is to come, the beauty beneath the surface. It's all a matter of perspective. Even in death, there is beauty.

Transformation Key: Perspective is a powerful tool, learn to become a master of perspective and observe the world from multiple viewpoints for it will serve you well.

46

15 November 2021: I Was Wiped Out

I was wiped out.

After a weekend of walking in the beautiful Autumn trees, I woke up this morning and decided I should do my physio workout.

Sheez that was harder than expected.

During the exercises I broke down and cried, I was so frustrated with the state that this f...ing stroke has left me in. I know I'm alive and I'm beyond grateful for that but I cannot help but get so frustrated with the inability to do basic things and/or activities that I used to do with ease. Sometimes I want to shout to God and say "WTF, why did you do this? Did you really think I wanted this?"

...and I know that the answer is Yes, for the universe/God/

Source Energy/Divine Intelligence (whatever name you like) only delivers what we've been energetically asking for! So at some twisted level, this was for me and it didn't happen to me ....I keep telling myself that so that I can somehow spiritually reconcile all this mess.

But, my human is pissed off in one almighty way. There are days when that comes out. There are days when my human self wants to scream and shout and find someone or something to blame, but my soul self wants to laugh at that behaviour and reminds me that God sent me this stroke to literally knock me off my feet... to make me stop like nothing has ever done before. I was running my life on overdrive constantly worried about everything.

After I finished and had breakfast my human self couldn't help but fall asleep for hours during the morning following this physio workout session....I think 2.5 - 3 hours extra sleep in a chair....sheez who knew that a few exercises could have such an impact?!

So onwards and upwards we go. The start of week 10 since the stroke occurred, recovery continues. And I am so grateful that recovery can continue but it doesn't mean that some days are not hard!

It's completely normal to feel crap after such a massive life-changing event such as a stroke or brain injury. There were days when I just wanted to shout and blame someone, anyone, anything, God, you name it, I wanted to blame something as a means of making myself somehow feel better about the situation. But the truth is, no one or nothing (no thing) is truly to blame, the situation has occurred and it was for me. I was deeply grateful for the opportunity to still live, but, of course, life would be different from now on.

Claire has taught me some deep spiritual-based healing work and that work has led me to understand that everything happens for us, not to us. That concept is hard to grasp, and the standard human reaction to anyone suggesting that having a brain haemorrhage was for them rather than it happening to them would be to say "Up yours mate!"

I understand that reaction, I truly do, but I've learned that being the witness to my condition helped me rise above the victim mode and move into a space of reconciliation about the situation.

I have subsequently come to hold a belief that God / Source Energy / Divine Intelligence (all the same thing to me) wants to experience through the human experience, and that experience has no bounds. God wants to experience everything through us (humans), God does not judge an experience as good or bad, it just is. So in that sense, a stroke is just an experience. To the human (me in this case) it's a shit experience, but to God, it's just an experience. I can imagine God saying, "I wonder what it's like to recover from brain damage?" and then going on to say, " I know, this bloke is fit and healthy enough to survive it. I don't want to kill the human involved in the experience or else I won't get to experience anything else from that human, I do not wish to destroy; I only create."

Another way, to look at it is that it happened for me as a result of a subconscious manifestation of the same frequency. What I mean by this is we create our own manifested reality and in that way, my entire life of thoughts and feelings will have thrown countless energetic frequencies out into the spiritual universe. Those frequencies find their match and come back to us in one lifetime or another. In that sense, the stroke might have even been an energetic frequency from a previous life. Think of it like a sound echoing back. The energy goes out and then it returns later. Get your head around that one!!

This might all sound strange to many people but I believe there is a reason for everything. Nothing in this universe happens by accident. There is a vast intelligence in spiritual mind that is creating everything and we (humans) are an integral part of that intelligence because we also create with our minds and our thoughts. In that sense, we are all God. Now get your head around that one!! I'm on a roll here.

But with all that said, the poor old human (in this case that is me) at the centre of the experience would sometimes wish that I was not the centre of the experience. However, remembering that it was part of a greater experience that I would learn from and go on to help others propelled me to surrender to what was happening and accept my situation with grace.

Transformation Key: When circumstances give you a rough hand, rather than playing the victim, adopt a sense of the "bigger picture". Move to a perspective of this happening for me and not to me.

47

16 November 2021: Duality

There is a common theme about this week 10 of my recovery.

I notice that I have a foot in either camp of immense frustration and immense gratitude.

Frustration with just about everything and anything, even frustration with life itself and my faith is being put to the test like never before. I've experienced many scenarios that have tested my faith, but none more so than this experience of being stripped of my abilities to earn a living, drive, to function without experiencing continuous imbalance.

Simultaneously, I have a foot in the camp of immense gratitude. Gratitude for all the love and support I am receiving day after day from Claire. Her unconditional love is truly immense and I will never take that for granted. The sight of the autumnal trees is truly breathtaking, the beauty of nature is incredible. Of course, I am so grateful to be alive, it really is a miracle that I'm here at all.

As I sit here in the car waiting in a local superstore car park, I ponder and ask myself "What is all of this for?"

As I mentally straddle this fine line between frustration and gratitude, I hope to God that I get to spend more time on the gratitude side rather than the side of frustration.

I acknowledge you frustration, I know you're there, I feel you, OMG I really feel you!!

But I yearn for you Gratitude, you are my saviour, you free me from turmoil and despair, and you provide me much-needed connection with my higher self.

As previously stated, the balance between my human ego-based self that wanted to scream and shout would be tempered by my more spiritual self that sought some form of spiritual meaning to my situation. It was a constant battle and I believe this period in November was when I started to notice that battle inside of myself.

Frustration vs. Gratitude was how I summed it up at the time. My human would get into deep frustration with the situation. It would cause great anguish that teetered on the edge of depression but I would be able to pull myself back by finding immense gratitude for still being alive, the continuous love from Claire and my ability to start to experience the world again.

This type of internal battle can easily become all-consuming and it is very easy to slip into a deep trough of low-frequency energy. The density of mood can be dangerously overpowering. If not kept in check, the side of frustration can take hold and it's easy to slip into a very depressed state.

Don't go there Find gratitude for anything

If you find that battle starts to rage inside of you. You might feel frustration in one moment and then immense gratitude the next. They seem to work against one another but my advice is to get behind gratitude every time. Frustration is a negative emotion and, whilst completely understandable, frustration will ultimately take you into a worse place mentally and emotionally, whereas gratitude allows you to see the world more positively and optimistically.

Transformation Key: Always look for gratitude in anything when the chips are down. Gratitude helps lift a mood to a higher frequency.

48

18 November 2021: Paddling Upstream

All my life I've been paddling upstream against the current. Of course, I didn't know that and it would result in behaviours that were based on achieving goals and striving for the next thing.

The Universe had other plans. Having the stroke literally knocked me off my feet. Now I find it so easy to slip into the void. That place of nothingness from where endless possibilities can arise.

Wow, that's exciting - endless possibilities!!

Whilst I can pine for the lost ability to focus on targets and goals, I could take a new approach that allows the possibilities to unfold.

I now know which approach works better for my entire physical,

> *mental and emotional well-being.*
> *Let's see what unfolds*

As I look back on my posts from mid-November 2021, I can see that was the time when I felt my spiritual awakening taking hold. It's interesting to observe the tension between my old human self and my newer spiritual self. The human self wanted to put up a fight, but the spiritual self was taking over.

I have read many books by some brilliant minds that have all played a part in this awakening along with my own beliefs. Dr Joe Dispenza has been an inspiration to me with his research into the power of the mind and deep meditation-based physical healing, his book Becoming Superhuman is a masterpiece. I recommend checking out his appearances on YouTube as well for some short introductions to him and his work. I think all of the reading and studying that I did pre-stroke laid the groundwork for this period.

I believe that we and everything else in the universe is energy and we are 'governed' by a source energy that is like the mounding clay of spiritual mind (a vast intelligence) that controls everything through thought. That vast soup of possibilities (unlimited thought) allows us (humans) as creative beings to create our reality. Whilst we have immense power through our thoughts to create whatever reality we desire, we are also influenced by the thoughts of others and the almost infinite number of thoughts that have ever been thought. This means that whilst anything is possible, we are also subject to other thoughts. Our reality is whatever we want to make it, and it all starts in the mind. Wow, we are so powerful.

As I pondered these ideas, I realised that I was leaving the old me behind more and more. I didn't know where this journey would take me but I surrendered to the journey whilst simultaneously envisioning my future in my thoughts. I balanced surrender and unfolding with thought and deliberate action to think and create my future whilst having the grace to let aspects of my new self gently unfold rather than force it into existence. This was happening whilst simultaneously I was allowing aspects of my old self to fall away. This was transformation.

Transformation Key: Everything is created in the mind through thought. We can think negatively and let fear and doubt dominate our thoughts, or we can think positively and let our imagination paint a picture of what we desire on the screen of our mind. We are always at choice how we think.

49

◈

21 November 2021: Losing Myself

Losing Myself

It's been ages since I lost myself playing a guitar!

Today I picked up one of my favourite guitars.

I've always just jammed and riffed out not following anything that anyone else knows.

One day I really should learn something that other people recognise....one day.

This morning, as I played, all my symptoms disappeared, no dizziness, no imbalance, no nausea, it was truly magical, I was momentarily transported to a different place where normality had been restored...it was bliss!

I taught myself the guitar when I was 13. I picked up my

Dad's nylon and steel-strung acoustic guitar. It was awful, but it was better than nothing and with a chord book in hand, I taught myself some basic chords. At 14 I spent some money that my Grandad had left me in his will and much to the neighbour's frustration, I bought myself an electric guitar and practice amp.

At 16 I left school and started an engineering apprenticeship so I then went to Stroud Technical College (later to become part of the University of Gloucester). I met Paul and Dave and, after a few years, we were all introduced to Lloyd. We had started to jam together and later formed a band, named Just. For a while, Marc (my mate from school) joined us too and then we had two drummers. It was a mad, noisy time with the battle of the drummers, electric guitar, bass, keyboards and vocals. Every practice session would result in ringing ears, getting stoned on hash and volume that would gradually increase, they were crazy times, but great memories.

We spent several years playing gigs and recording in various studios. It was a good period of my life which I look back on fondly. Tragically, Dave died in a motorcycle accident. Shortly after, I was blessed with my first child, Bryony. Not long following the birth of Bryony I decided my taste for band life had run its course and family life became my reality. But despite leaving Just, I still liked to pick up the guitar for my own (and my children's) amusement.

So, on that day in November 2021, I recall sitting on the bed and looking at my favourite acoustic guitar. It is a cheap thing but it plays well. At that time in my recovery I was still feeling nauseous with the dizziness and imbalance; it was a constant feeling that never went away.

Lo and behold, when I picked up the guitar and started to play, the nausea feeling stopped. As I played, I picked up the rhythm and got into a driving, rhythmic riff. In that moment of pure flow, all my symptoms went away. No dizziness, no awareness of imbalance and no nausea. My brain had finally, just for a moment, allowed me to experience life with a sense of normality again. It was fleeting, but it had happened. There was hope. I realised that I could return to a state of normality again. In that short period, I realised that my brain could re-member how to be a normal fully developed brain again. Full recovery might take a moment or it might take a moment, there was no telling how long that moment might take. But that didn't matter to me because I had been given the taste of normality again. Moreover, my brain had shown me that it knew how to be "normal" again. In that moment I knew for certain that I could fully recover. It might take a split second, minutes, hours, days, months, years or the rest of my life on earth. It will take what it will take. That was all I needed to keep me going.

We often dismiss the incredible power of flow. Flow is when we experience time standing still and we "lose ourselves" in the pursuit of a creative experience whether that is playing a musical instrument, writing, drawing, painting, martial arts, yoga, meditation or countless other experiences. When we reach a state of flow, resistance in our mind and negative emotions held in the body mind can dissipate which makes way for new neurology to be formed and new possibilities to be thought of and imagined. It is common for people experiencing flow to experience the "eureka moment" for great innovations and ideas. Flow is extremely powerful and transformative.

Transformation Key: Get into your flow. Achieving the flow state can unlock all manner of possibilities for personal transformation.

50

21 November 2021:
Cooking

> Cooking
> *Happy to be back in the cooking driving seat today!!*

I have always enjoyed cooking meals for Claire and the family; I feel a great sense of achievement from following a new recipe or cooking up a family favourite.

One of the signs of my continued recovery would be taking on the task of cooking a meal for the family. This is not a small task with two households totalling eight people (Claire, me, 4 children and Claire's parents Anita and Roger). A typical Sunday roast requires the peeling of a lot of potatoes for roasting, then multiple vegetables perhaps broccoli, carrots, peas etc., and then there is the roast itself and gravy.

As anyone who has cooked a large roast dinner can testify, creating a great roast is all about timing. Well for my recovering stroke brain, timing and remembering multiple boiling saucepans, and numerous other tasks was quite a challenge, believe me.

But, in typical fashion, I was determined. I wanted to be normal again and I wanted to show all the family that I could do it. I can't lie, it was very hard. I've subsequently recognised and admitted that maybe trying to cook a roast dinner for eight with a recovering brain injury was a lot harder than expected.

I remember on another occasion when we decided to cook Swede mashed with Carrot, that it all went wrong and I had to ask Claire to rescue the dinner for us all. I knew that Swede took a long time to boil and soften so I put the Swede on to cook far too early. That resulted in the Swede and Carrot mash being ready to serve before anything else was cooked! Oops! It's interesting, my brain knew that there was a timing exception in the form of Swede that takes a long time to cook, but my brain then clearly couldn't work out what adaptations had to occur with the rest of the cooking to incorporate the exception.

This is representative of a common theme as I've recovered. My ability to multi-task has been severely diminished. I'm not worrying about it too much because I know everything will return in time, and if not then that's ok too. There was a time in my recovery when not being able to multi-task and making a mistake with the cooking due to Swede might have made me upset and frustrated with myself. Now I've learnt to 'let it go'. If I can't do something for now, I accept it, admit it to others and move on.

Transformation Key: Let go of stuff that doesn't serve your transformation. Learn to laugh at yourself. Be kind to yourself.

51

22 November 2021: Celebrating

Celebrating

Over the past few weeks, my blood pressure has been stabilising! I've been doing a lot of work (both inner as well as outer work) to lead a more mindfully based lifestyle, living in the present rather than constantly worrying about the future or concerning myself with what others might think of me.

I've had to let a lot of things go, I had previously been holding onto things that actually I had to let go of and trust that the universe had everything covered for the highest good of all. That was scary but freedom was waiting for me on the other side all along. I just had to trust and face the fear

Freedom from the continuous torture of the mind - the kind of torture that leads to stress and high blood pressure!

Every day I start my day with measuring my BP and I've witnessed the outer (the measurement) getting closer and closer to the target set by the docs in the hospital about 8 weeks ago. That target was 130/80

Today the 7 day average was:

130/87.

Almost there!! So today I'm celebrating my own personal wins.

I'm celebrating mindfulness

I'm celebrating letting go

I'm celebrating trust in the universe

I'm celebrating my belief in my daily meds

I'm celebrating my approach that embraces all modalities - from scientific to ancient to esoteric

Celebrating wins is so important to achieve a long-term goal and objective.

I believe that we have two ultimately powerful creative forces that reside within us. We have a force for good and creation and an opposing force for destruction. Celebrating wins helps combat the force of destruction and fear. This destructive force that is based upon fear creates feelings of doubt and insecurity within us. If left unchecked, those doubts, insecurities, worries, and concerns will take hold of our creative path and cause us to lose our way. I imagine a flowerbed sown with seeds of pretty flowers and then along come the weeds to strangle out the sprouting flowers. If left unchecked, the flowerbed will just become a bed of tangled weeds.

When my doctors were treating me in the hospital they stated that my target blood pressure should be 130/80 and they set me on a course of prescription medication aimed at achieving and supporting that target.

It probably doesn't come as much surprise that I now carefully monitor my blood pressure. Following the advice of my GP, I monitor my blood pressure regularly using a monitor designed with an upper arm cuff. I am told that these give a more accurate reading than the other general-purpose wrist-worn devices that measure pulse etc.

My blood pressure does fluctuate and I've now noticed that certain situations can cause it to rise quite significantly. For instance, conflict seems to have a detrimental effect on my blood pressure. One of the interesting factors is also how the blood pressure is quick to rise but can be extremely slow to drop or stabilise again. A situation occurred recently (within the last month) that caused a significant rise but then it wouldn't drop down again. It rose to the 150/100 types of levels (not healthy) and yet my medication was the same as before. I recognised that I had experienced some personal conflict which upset me. Whilst my body felt okay, the monitoring of my blood pressure told me that my body was still experiencing the after-effects of the conflict. It makes me think that we don't appreciate what stresses we put ourselves under when we experience conflict or upset in our daily lives.

I'm pleased to say that intervention with an additional medicine along with a change of mindset and various changes in diet helped create a more stabilised daily blood pressure reading of 125/84. My personal goal for my blood pressure is 127/78.

Transformation Key: Put all your thought energy into your future vision and let thoughts based on fear and doubt pass through your mind without attachment or meaning. Both types of thoughts will create.

52

23 November 2021: Giving Up The Worry

Giving up the Worry.
As I work through this season of my life I've come to realise that the most beneficial thing I can do is give up worrying about stuff.
I've been a worrier all my life:
From the big stuff like:

Money
Relationships
Health

To the small stuff like:

Gifts

Making the "right" impression

Things that could spill or cause a mishap ...and a million other micro-things!!

...and I wondered why I have Hypertension !!?? Sheez it's no wonder I have Hypertension!!!

So, in these last 10 weeks of stroke recovery, probably the biggest of all recoveries is facing my fears and walking right up to each one as I work through my incessant fixation with worry!!

The irony is that in order to combat worry, worry itself has to not be a thing! Wow, get your head around that!

So please wish me luck as I embark on creating this new version of me

As this post states, I have been an insentient worrier pretty much all my life! This is not healthy at all. It is only when I reflect on my life journey that I release the extent of my fixation on worry. I would worry about pretty much anything, to be honest.

A large part of the redemptive transformation of my whole self has been this realisation and when I think about it more I wonder if being a worry addict has been a big part of the cause of my hypertension.

The root cause of worry is fear and a deep sense of not being good enough. Many people are afflicted by this suffering and it is entirely constructed in the ego-mind as an exaggerated form of protection. In other words, it is the ego-mind's over-exuberant efforts to keep everyone separate. Again, in other words, it's made up! We make this sh!t up in our minds and none of it is true. How completely insane is that?

The antidote for this form of suffering is to let yourself feel the light and love in the heart. That is easier said than done though. How do we feel the light and love from the heart when the addiction to worry and self-loathing is so strong? The ego-mind is such a strong opponent and we often convince ourselves that we're not good enough for this, not good enough for that, and on and on we go. It is all BS!

Awareness is the first key to this healing. Becoming aware and admitting the addiction is the first step in any recovery of a spiritual nature. Don't judge the addiction to worry and not being good enough. You are not alone. Really! You are not alone in this suffering.

Become aware that this is just a thing but don't be tempted to give it meaning or give it a label. Just learn to be the witness of the addiction and learn to say, "Aha, I see you." and then hear yourself say "I love you". This might bring up tears and emotions and that is ok too; think of the tears as helping to wash away the pain and suffering from the addiction to worry and self-loathing, but nothing more. In my own experience, as I pass through this healing (it's happened several times), I reach a point where I shut my eyes, take a deep breath and hear the words in myself, "I love you." These words are repeated over and over again as I feel a deep feeling of calm and peace wash over me as the realisation of being good enough is already known deep within us all.

I like to think of the situation like this; being born into this human experience is so rare and improbable within the context of the massiveness of the universe that it follows that we are all so worthy to even exist at all. Ok, that is big... I get it. Too big for me to explain perhaps. It is inexplicable. But I think that's the point. I, you, us, we are so unbelievably worthy to have this opportunity to experience life on earth that we are completely good enough just as we are.

Worrying is so pointless. Feelings of self-loathing and not being good enough are utterly pointless. We are all totally good enough just exactly as we are; probably more than we'll ever truly and deeply understand during this life experience.

We are all good enough just as we are. When you look into your heart and relax into the love that emanates from that space you can hear a whisper that you know is the sound of your higher self saying to you that you are perfect; you are worthy; you are more than enough; you are God.

Transformation Key: You were born worthy.

53

⟨❈⟩

2 December 2021: Recovery Update

Recovery Update

It's almost 12 weeks since I survived my brain haemorrhage (stroke).

There are days when that time has dragged and there are days when it's flown by.

One thing I've tried to sustain throughout my recovery and into the future is a sense of positivity and optimism. I've avoided using words like victim or suffered as these tend to make me think in a negative way.

One of the targets I set myself shortly after the stroke was to return to the rugby club to stand pitch side and watch my son training or playing in his U13s group.

Last night Claire drove my son and I to the club and together

> (Claire and I) we were able to watch him training .... Yay! Super happy about that
> The future's looking good!

It is very easy to be the victim of life. We think that being the victim seems to serve us at some twisted level, but it doesn't. I'm sorry if that sounds harsh, but maybe it needs to be harsh to help break free of that warped illusion.

When I stagger around and can't think straight, or I have to think hard to tie my shoelaces properly or have to re-focus every time I perform my yoga routines, I could easily fall into victim mode and ask, "Why me?" and "It's not fair." That would be easy. The harder thing to do is to set goals and visions for a future where all those things are once again, just second nature to a fully functioning and healthy brain. It's hard when the current reality appears so far away from the goal or the vision.

But who says that having to refocus before doing a yoga pose is wrong anyway? Maybe that's normal? Maybe having to concentrate on tying shoelaces is a thing. It's a complex task for any brain to figure out, so having to relearn these things is just part of the opportunity to start over again; it's all part of my transformation.

I've talked about the importance of setting goals and visions in other parts of this book. Every aspect of recovery and transformation has an element of goal setting and vision incorporated within it.

Having goals and a vision is the first part of any transformation whether that's associated with a recovery from Stroke or not. The act of experiencing the vision of the goal achieved means that in some universal dimension, it has already happened. For our human ego mind that seems illogical but is it? I don't think so. In my worldview, I like to think that if I can experience the vision, then it is just a matter of which reality I choose to make the truth; the reality where I'm still recovering or the reality where I am already recovered.

To help me choose, my human ego-mind needs to see results to continue on the path of recovery. So then I take aligned action to fulfil that vision. It might take a significant amount of action and repetition or it may happen instantly; after all, time is a human-made concept. Our 12-month calendar came about because of two Roman emperors, Julius Caesar and Augustus (July and August). What we are also referring to is faith and belief. Having faith and belief when the current reality is contrary to that faith and belief is hard. But it is possible.

One of my favourite things to do is watch my son play rugby. I recall when I was in the hospital just after the stroke I said to Claire, and my physiotherapy team, that I wanted to get back to watching him practice and play rugby at the club.

12 weeks later, I returned to the club to watch him practice on

a very cold, Wednesday evening. Poor Claire had to endure so much as we rebuilt my life.

Transformation Key: When you experience a vision for your future it is like peering through a hole in time. Your current reality may not reflect that vision but at all times you have a choice of where to focus your energy. Do you focus on the current reality or do you focus on making your vision your reality?

54

6 December 2021: I Ran

I RAN!!

We had to get out for a walk! The dark clouds that had been building on the horizon were now directly overhead. It was obvious that the rain was going to start at any time, but still we went anyway.

As we climbed the first stile into the fields, we felt the first blobs of rain; large and heavy. The wind grew stronger; cold and wild. We were exposed to the weather by being in the field; there was no protection anywhere; we were going to get soaked!!

The only protection was on the other side of the large hedge but the access point was halfway up the length of the field.... there was nothing else;no other option..... RUN!!!

Running in a field, wearing a large coat, welly boots, scarf, hat and gloves in the howling wind and rain is not an easy task....try adding stroke recovery into the mix as well!!! F..k!

It was amazing. I felt alive. Yes, everything was wobbly in my head, but I did it. I stayed on my feet! I ran across the field! For some, you might say so what but to me this was monumental.

As I start week 13 of my recovery from the brain haemorrhage I would never have imagined that I'd be running.

We ran to the gap in the hedge, crossed into the shelter and calm. Soon the rain passed and we had amazing views of the sun and clouds before sunset and we were able to walk the woods and back into the field.

Fun times!!

Today has been a good day

Sometimes, the universe will throw a situation in your way that is sent to test you once again.

These tests might be large or small. These tests will make you question the next immediate move. Should I do it or should I back away? My advice is to listen to your heart at that moment. If it says no way and that resistance is associated with a loving feeling then maybe it's not the right time to do 'the thing'. If there's excitement and there's a loving pull to just do it, then do it!

The human ego-mind will always want to protect you (which is a good thing and stops you walking straight into danger) but it can also make us over-think things and prevent us from experiencing the thrill of life. Sometimes the right thing to do is feel the freedom and pull of the heart.

This post from early December 2021 was one of those moments.

The late months of 2021 were an exceptionally difficult time for the family. We experienced so many challenges that resulted in my recovery being reprioritised and pushed down the list of priorities. At the time that felt hard to accept but I had no choice and as my physiotherapist at the time (Alice) said to me, "Being priority 4 is a good thing and is a reflection on how well you are recovering." That was probably the best advice I could have received from anyone at that time.

So there we were in that moment walking in the fields on that Winters day and then the cold rain came down, accompanied by strong winds. We had a choice to make, turn back and try to find some shelter or run to the point where we could cut through the hedge and shelter behind the large hedge. At that moment, turning back was not an option; I didn't even consider it. So we ran.

It was a much-needed moment of joy, which in itself was a relief from all the craziness of our lives during that time.

Transformation Key: "Feel the fear and do it anyway" is a well-known phrase that plays out in our lives all the time. You will know in your heart when the fear and danger is real or not. Don't let the ego-mind-created fear stop you from experiencing the joy of the moment.

55

6 December 2021: Happy
Happy Happy

Happy Happy Happy

This morning I had my lowest blood pressure reading since my stroke.

I am over the moon right now!!!

As a family, we are going through so much at the moment. Everything is being thrown at us. The stroke that I had 12+ weeks ago is only part of the story!

It is in these types of trials that we are truly tested. Tested on every level. Physically; emotionally; mentally; financially; and spiritually.

In the past, this level of trial could easily manifest in my body as stupidly high blood pressure.

The underlying cause of my brain haemorrhage was hypertension and high blood pressure. So avoiding stress is imperative but stress is everywhere; it's impossible to avoid; in fact, the avoidance of stress is itself...stressful! Doh

So this morning's reading of 122/82 feels amazing to me. Whilst science and meds have contributed, I know that the primary factor to this great reading is mindset.

Some mornings (not today) my readings might start in the 150's so I breathe. I breathe into my body and visualise a reading in the 120's; I generate the feeling of what under 130 feels like to me; safe; calm; stable...and then hey presto, the reading drops accordingly. The power we have over our own state is amazing. It's a matter of belief!! I now eat stress for breakfast.

Have a great day

The power of the mind and our thoughts to create our reality is the most important factor in any recovery or transformation.

We often forget this vital component to our detriment. It is not just the power of thought, it is the associated feeling of the thought and vision fulfilled that holds the secret. The feeling comes from the heart, and it is the magnetic power of the heart that attracts the results we seek. It is so easy to slip off the "good-feeling" wagon and return to a default position of allowing thinking (and feeling) the worst to dominate.

As stated so many times in this book, we are always at choice about how we choose to think and feel. It is the endless human struggle. Which thoughts, which inner voice and which feelings are we going to choose? Which feelings are we allowing to dominate?

The same amount of energy is required for both choices but thinking, feeling and acting with thoughts and feelings that come from a place of fear result in us taking action based on fear and the resultant creation will be far, far away from our desires. It is by thinking, feeling and taking action based on creating our desired outcomes that build the results that we seek.

There is no denying it, making the right choice is hard. But ultimately the choice is ours and ours alone to make. No one can choose for us.

Transformation Key: We are always at choice with where we expend our thought, feeling and action energy. It is when we channel that energy towards our desired outcomes that we start to build the life we seek.

56

~~~~~

8 December 2021:
Balancing

BALANCING

Ever since I survived the stroke (brain haemorrhage) 12.5 weeks ago I've been feeling drunk due to the brain damage in my cerebellum.

The cerebellum in the brain controls many things including balance.

Every day for the past week and into the foreseeable future I have to do what I call "my head exercises".

4 times a day I lie on my bed and turn my head right then left. This brings on the drunk symptoms (especially turning left).

Once the symptoms start I then stop and let my head and body recover (typically under 0.5sec at the moment).

The purpose is to build new neurology to replace the damage.

> *Stroke and recovery (if you're lucky to survive) are very real. My stroke was caused by hypertension and high blood pressure...which was caused by stress. I used to get anxious about the smallest and biggest of things!*
>
> *If you get stressed and anxious let's chat. I would hate for this to happen to anyone else!*
>
> *Be kind to yourself*

Small steps will lead you to accomplish great feats.

The feeling of imbalance was and is a primary feature of the Cerebellar Stroke that I experienced. The imbalance is a result of the brain damage that occurred when the haemorrhage happened. The 4cm patch of brain in my brain caused the brain tissue in that area of my brain to die.

As explained to me and as explained before in this book, the brain will replace and build new neural networks to replace damaged neurology. This is called neuroplasticity and it's incredible!

To help me rebuild the neurology to help my balance, associated nausea and unbelievable feelings of dizziness, I had to undertake various exercises day after day.

My physiotherapy nurse, Alice, devised a simple head-turning plan to specifically invoke the dizziness, imbalance and nausea. It was pretty grim and it felt pointless at the time but doing the things you don't want to do is part of the healing and recovery process. Just suck it up (metaphorically) and get on with it!

I might sound harsh but once again, this is about choice and deciding which actions are going to help towards achieving the ultimate goal.

In typical fashion for me, I soon mixed the head bed exercises up a bit and eventually turned that into my morning and evening yoga/pilates/strength training routine. If I felt it was necessary to return to the head-bed exercises I would in an instant. The process of moving and twisting my head on the bed was a vital part of building the neurology needed to navigate the world around me.

Transformation Key: Sometimes we have to do the thing we don't want to. We might be bored, or we might feel ill, or we might get frustrated with the time it takes to see any results, Stick with it! The transformation will take time. The amount of time is unknown so we just have to stick with the plan. To ease the monotony keep a record of results to chart progress.
When we see small incremental improvements it helps us stay the course.

57

9 December 2021: Don't Look Up

DON'T LOOK UP!

I was walking Toby our dog and I heard the sound of a small(ish) aircraft. The engine tone was increasing and decreasing as it climbed and descended in the sky.

My intrigue got the better of me so I looked up into the sky.

Oh boy, that was weird!!

I felt the strain on my shins as my body wanted to topple over as my balance completely went. My head spun wildly.

"Mmm, weird", I thought to myself, "let's try that again"....

No, definitely not a good idea. The head spinning and utter disorientation dominated my body. It felt like I was hanging upside down...proper weird!!!

I think that had I persisted I would have ended up flat on my face in the middle of the field

Here's my learning from that experience.... I need references as I'm looking around. The sky was just an endless grey cloud (typical crappy UK sky). Nothing to distinguish near from far or any sense of perspective, just empty nothingness.
My balance skills are shot to shit anyway, but add an endless boring grey nothingness in the mix and wow, it's all over!! Close to face plant!
Have a great day

Sometimes it's not a great idea to do things that are difficult on any given day, let alone when we're going through a challenging time. But there is something that can be taken from every experience, including those that don't deliver the best outcome.

When we realise that every moment of our lives is to experience and learn then everything we do, or every situation we experience is there to teach us something. We often think that situations happen to us. I disagree. Everything happens for us. I believe we create our experiences and therefore our reality, even the aspects of life that appear to the human ego-mind as being challenging and upsetting. We create it all and we create it all for a purpose.

I believe that we attract into our life experience that which we emanate. We project energy because that is exactly what we are. We are energy vibrating in a vast range of frequencies.

The brain is the incredible supercomputer that interprets all of the energy detected by our senses. What we see, hear, smell, taste and touch. Although there is no seeing as such, it's the optic nerve and associated systems of nerves and neurology that translate light energy in our brains into images in the mind and that light energy enters our bodies through our eyes. We interpret the images as something (e.g. an aeroplane in the sky) and we give it a name (which is recalled from memory) and we hear (sound energy) through our ears and the brain interprets that sound as the engine and associates the aeroplane with the sound and hey presto we enrich the experience. But this is all energy (e.g. light and sound in this example) interacting with energy (me, my brain etc.)

Everything we experience is through forms of energy interpreted by the brain, the ego-mind, the heart, our life force, the body-mind, our memories, our conditioning, our beliefs and all of those around us (more and more energy systems). We literally "make up" our entire life experience through an interpretation with all of these filters, and almost 9 billion of us are constantly doing this on this spaceship called planet Earth.

When put like that, it's quite something, isn't it!?! That is probably the biggest understatement ever written by anyone, anywhere! It's way more than just 'quite something'! And people still question the existence of vast intelligence and a universal life force. Oh well, I guess some will always do that.

When we experience something that we think doesn't serve

us, at some deeper level it probably does. One of the many filtering systems that help us make up our world might well be orchestrating a series of events for its (and therefore our) own benefit.

This might have been the case when I looked up into the sky to try to find the looping aeroplane. The experience caused me to almost topple over but I learnt something from the experience. To most people, the idea of tilting one's head back to look into a featureless blank sky would almost always result in imbalance and dizziness and then induce a sense of falling, but to my life experience and in my state of re-learning and rebooting my life, it was a new learning experience. It was something I had to learn for myself in that moment.

This reminds me of another aspect of my life which is my human design. For those reading this that have an awareness of human design, I am a manifesting generator with a 1:3 profile. The 1:3 profile defines an aspect of my life which is categorised using the archetypes of The Investigator and The Martyr. The Martyr is characterised as having experiential learning traits and one who only learns through experience.

Transformation Key: We are here to learn from experience. In some, this may be a recurring aspect of life. Our experiences teach us and help us grow into better versions of ourselves. The experiences are always for us at some level, the experiences never happen to us.

58

11 December 2021: Driving

DRIVING

I'm driving again!!!!

Omg, this is massive news.

So late yesterday afternoon, as it was getting dark, Claire and I realised that we needed to shop for the weekend groceries and drop off my son's cleaned rugby kit at his mum's for the weekend.

"Do you want to drive?", Claire asked slightly nervously.

"Yes!", I replied confidently.

So with that, I jumped into the driver's side, and Claire into the passenger side and away we went!

First time in 13 weeks!

I've been very hesitant up to now to even consider driving. Having a persistent feeling of drunkenness does not lend itself to driving....at all.

But here's the weird thing, when I drive, play the guitar or sit and do something creative or distracting, the drunken feeling goes away. It only comes back when I stand or walk.

If I walk around I stagger (sometimes a little, sometimes a lot)...people who don't know what has happened to me, give me a look of...drunken fool! It's not great I must admit.

Anyway, back to driving. I drove us to the supermarket and then to drop off the rugby kit....and we made it! It was dark, the road was busy, there were a lot of lights, thin roads, our vehicle is big (VW Transporter 9 seater shuttle....its a bus!)...and we made it without a hitch.....

So here's to another huge milestone in my recovery.

I love driving, I always have done. It was a huge milestone to start driving again although driving the large VW Transporter Shuttle (bus) took a lot of concentration, I can tell you, and that resulted in my increased brain fatigue, but I had done it!

One could be forgiven for thinking that driving when I had a continuous feeling of being dizzy and imbalanced was not a very sensible idea. I would have agreed, but the interesting phenomenon I discovered was that all symptoms of dizziness and imbalance went away immediately. I was focused and could work all the necessary multi-tasking elements of driving without any problem at all.

I think stretching myself to do things that were previously not possible helped to increase the pace of my recovery. It felt really good to take on these, formerly, normal tasks, such as driving.

For 13 weeks prior, Claire had been our primary driver but her ankle had started to get aggravated by the clutch pedal on the bus. She had taken over as the primary driver of our family ever since the previous September 11th when she drove us all home from the rugby festival with me lying in the back of the bus with a brain haemorrhage. Here we were on December 11th, exactly 3 months later, and I was able to drive the bus again... that was super fast in terms of the pace of recovery.

Transformation Key: Sometimes you can stretch yourself to reach heights that just a few moments earlier (hours, days, weeks, months) seemed impossible. There's a saying, "Leap and you'll grow wings". When the time is right, and you'll know it deep within you, then take that leap!

59

14 December 2021: Square Peg - Round Hole

SQUARE PEG - ROUND HOLE

For all my adult life I've felt out of place. During my recovery from stroke (in week 14 now), I've been led to research neuro-diversity and I've discovered that I have moderate autism. I've had this all my adult life and it led to me having to pretend to be someone I wasn't (almost a double life!!) just to fit in.

Living a double life created so much stress for me. I piled on every other "normal" stress; money; divorce; children; aspirations; career; etc., but being a square peg in a round hole was awful. I was a mess.

That stress manifested itself in high blood pressure which then almost killed me. I ignored the warning signs thinking I knew best. I didn't... then a brain haemorrhage

> *STOP! Everything stopped.*
> *Please don't ignore the warning signs. If you want help, DM me.*

I started to research Neurodiversity because we had a family member showing traits of ASD (Autism Spectrum Disorder). These traits resulted in an incident that then led to an unfair and unwarranted permanent exclusion from school. It was yet another traumatic time for the family.

Understandably, Claire's attention was completely taken away from me and my recovery to focus on this latest challenge to family life. We had to quickly adapt to having another child permanently in the house with us as I was navigating recovery and Claire was balancing the family, the home, running her business, my recovery and now this latest delivery of chaos.

It felt like we were being tested from every possible direction. It was a very hard time for everyone in the family, but I suppose most of all, Claire. She must have been screaming inside. "Please universe, what next?" "No more tests please!"

As I did my part to help as best as I could, I researched ASD and I decided to take an online assessment that I had found. I carefully answered each multiple-choice question that related to different scenarios and I found to my astonishment that many of the scenarios and questions resonated deeply with me. I was cognisant to consider my responses about my former self and not be swayed by my current recovering self.

As I completed the assessment I reviewed the score and

outcome, and the assessment rated me as moderately autistic. It was a revelation to me and strangely, it felt like a relief. Finally, I felt recognised and I felt a sense of belonging after all this time (almost 54 years).

In my adult life, I had always felt like I never really fit in and at times it was a struggle to navigate professional and social settings without any anxiety or feelings of awkwardness. I had done a good job of masking my struggles, and in many respects, this had made the situation worse for me. The more people accepted me, the harder it seemed to be to keep up the masking. I didn't know who I was and I would be many personas. I made this mean there was something wrong or that I was wrong. It fed the lie that I had created that I wasn't good enough.

This is typical of the torture of the human ego mind. It wants to make us think we're separate from one another as a form of protection but the result is we feel utterly lost, desperate and alone; it's a serious mental condition that I believe can lead to anxiety, depression and suicidal ideation. I would also advocate that it can lead to extreme stress and hypertension. I have no proof of that association, it is just my theory, but I would wager that there is a direct link between undiagnosed ASD, stress and hypertension. Getting a formal diagnosis takes ages (18 months) so I didn't pursue that avenue. In my mind, I had read enough to feel a sense of relief.

I am not one for labels and I am aware that undertaking a self-diagnosis from an assessment on the internet could lead to a misdiagnosis but I didn't care about all that. Being moderately autistic and understanding the associated behavioural traits made complete sense to me; it was like a safe harbour for me; I felt like I was reading about myself.

Transformation Key: Understand who you are and stand in your truth. When we mask and hide who we are we create unhealthy stress and anxiety within us that leads us to question our self-worth. When we are truly authentic and have the confidence to stand whole-heartedly and unshakeable in the truth of who we are, we discover an inner power so strong that we permit others to shine in their truth too.

60

⚭

15 December 2021: I Surrender

I Surrender.

I've tried to 'push on' and I've made some huge strides in my recovery journey.

However, my recovery and this period of pause in my life have unearthed some deeper healing that I need to do.

I hold my hands up, "Yes guilty as charged", for constantly filling the void with distractions and external conditions, simply a means to avoid the silence within, and yet ironically I am seeking inner peace above everything else.

Peace from trauma, peace from self-doubt and feelings of unworthiness, peace from the chaos of life itself (our family is being tested from every possible direction at the moment).

So what can I really do in this moment?

Nothing!

So I surrender with trust and grace with an inner knowing that at some level this is all happening for us and not to us. I surrender so that in the silence I might learn the teaching, accept the healing, and move with the next nudge in a direction that is unknown and uncertain.

There is a term in business which (I believe) comes from the military, which I realise applies to life itself.

The term is VUCA - Volatility, Uncertainty, Complexity and Ambiguity. To not just survive but thrive with VUCA requires immense Resilience.

For some, resilience can come from a push energy, for me, in this moment, push has built resistance, so I choose to surrender.

Have a blessed day

Inner peace is my state of bliss. In my worldview, inner peace is the place that I can reach if I allow myself. To decide to reach for inner peace is a conscious one. I can easily get distracted by outside influences to draw my attention or give me that "hit" of momentary satisfaction, but in the end, none of the momentary "hits" can replace the deep euphoria of inner peace.

Part of the conscious effort to choose inner peace is not any effort at all. When there is effort involved then resistance builds which creates a blockage to inner peace, so the answer (for me) is a conscious surrender to the outside noise, turmoil and distractions. This level of surrendering takes great trust and resilience.

As I navigated this period of my recovery with all of the other challenges being thrown simultaneously at our family, I had no choice but to fully surrender. I had to just trust that the universe would have our back and that we would all be okay.

I cried so many times. I was frustrated that I couldn't do what I might have used to. I was frustrated that I had been stripped of my ability to think straight and figure out a way through. I felt useless. My human-ego mind was scared, hurt, and afraid. I had no other option but to surrender to the will of God and trust that everything would work out even though in that period it felt like everything was falling apart. I was so thankful that through all of the madness somehow Claire and I stayed together, although it truly tested our relationship to the max. There were no arguments, no shouting. I don't think I could have handled that as well, that would have sent my already shattered nervous system into complete self-destruction if that had happened too. We stayed strong.

It took so much resilience to navigate that period and all the challenges being thrown at us. I was recovering from a brain haemorrhage, one child had been self-harming as a result of mental health and anxiety, another child had been excluded from school and had un-diagnosed moderate ASD, Claire was trying to navigate schooling systems that had utterly failed us and trying to show up to market her coaching business, my parents were being admitted to hospital because of increasing dementia-related issues only to get pushed back home for the issues to happen again and again, Christmas was just around the corner, and we didn't know where the next money was coming from to pay the bills, let alone gifts for Christmas for the kids. It was an unbelievably difficult time. The pressure was immense. If anyone could teach about resilience, it's Claire and I as we metaphorically navigated a terrible storm at sea with vast waves that would crush our frail sailing boat containing our lives at any moment.

Transformation Key: Sometimes all you have is trust and faith. In the moments when everything seems lost it is possible to find resilience from a place of deep surrender, trust and faith. When nothing makes sense and the mind cannot fathom the solution(s) then that is the time when your resilience, trust and faith will be rewarded. You will somehow get through the storm!

61

16 December 2021: Coping With Stress

Coping with Stress

Sometimes it can feel as if nothing else could go wrong! The mounting pressure of stress from every possible angle can seem relentless. Whether it's huge life-changing events or smaller events, the build-up of stress can seem overwhelming.

For me, those stress factors resulted in high blood pressure which eventually triggered a brain hemorrhage (stroke).

Yet another rather stressful event, you might say!

Today, one of the best techniques I use to reduce my BP and stress is intentional deep breathing.

I should have done this years ago! My discovery is somewhat too late for me, but it doesn't need to be too late for you. I realise now, that I'd always known deep breathing, but I never really

> *took it seriously. I knew it academically, but I never embodied it properly.*
>
> *If you carry stress in your body; if you get high anxiety about any situation, then please try and embody this technique, it can have a huge benefit.*
>
> *Have a wonderful stress stress-free day*

Intentional deep breathing can have a positive effect on stress and the resulting conditions such as anxiety, and high blood pressure.

Whenever I feel tension in my body which will very often be in my chest, I take a lovely deep breath in through my nose and then gently blow it out through my mouth in a smooth circular motion. Even as I sit here typing these words I am doing it and I can feel the positive effects on my body and my brain. I can feel the tension lifting with each breath, it is wonderful.

I recall a moment during the latter months of 2021 when I disagreed with one of the kids. Our opposing viewpoints on a situation caused conflict to arise. I felt hurt and not heard regarding a situation where I was judged as being egotistical. This caused conflict to arise. I now acknowledge that I do not like conflict and it might have been a contributing factor to the spike in blood pressure and the haemorrhage itself; I suppose I'll never truly find out. That being said, when the conflict with one of the children occurred I could feel the tension in my body. My chest felt tight and my brain started to, what I only describe as, throb.

What this scenario brought to my attention was the detrimental effect of carrying old emotional wounding. It's interesting that where I felt I was judged and misunderstood, it triggered emotions buried deep within my body that then led to feelings of conflict arising within me. It is so important that we deal with our emotional wounding as we never know when or what might trigger us and cause us to act out of character or behave irrationally. Worse still, emotional wounds can lay dormant for months and years and then suddenly a trigger occurs and we feel the emotional response rise within us (anger, bitterness, frustration, sadness, fear, conflict etc.) To others, the response is deemed irrational and yet to us, the response is completely justified. The truth is we need to heal those old emotional wounds so that if/when the trigger scenario re-occurs it does not affect us at all. This trauma is a form of PTSD (Post Traumatic Stress Disorder) and is increasingly recognised as being present in many people.

When I felt the tension rise in me from the conflict I sensed the danger signals in my body (tight chest, throbbing brain etc.) We stopped the conflict and I took my blood pressure. Wow, it spiked dramatically to 190+ / 100+. This was very dangerous territory. The conflict ceased immediately. I can't remember how we resolved our differences now, but I do know that there were tears as we both realised and acknowledged just has damaging conflict can potentially be to one's health.

I started to breathe to bring my blood pressure down again. It took about 10 minutes of intentional deep breathing and eventually, my blood pressure reduced to 148/94. This is still not super safe blood pressure but it is a lot better than the excessive reading that I had taken 10 minutes earlier.

Transformation Key: Intentional deep breathing can have a dramatic positive effect on lowering and stabilising blood pressure. Never underestimate the power of breath on the body and mind.

62

◈

17 December 2021: Music

MUSIC.

It's time to get creative! I can lose myself for hours creating music...

I love it

Today I decided to dust off my MIDI controller, figured out my headphones (Bluetooth issue) and fired up GarageBand.

This is my happy place. The world might be falling apart around me but I'll just be blissfully unaware as the sounds in my ears take me to "a place".

Ok, I'm going to get back to it...

...laters

Being a musician, it probably won't be surprising that creating music sends me to my flow state. I tend to lose myself in the sounds that I'm playing with and more often than not, I don't end up creating anything decent as a result. This is the case when I play with my MIDI controller and looping software. The result will typically go one of two ways; I'll get into it and create a track that when I review it again later in the future, I'll either love or hate. The other route that might typically happen is that I will get lost or stuck in the technology and end up in a state of frustration and then switch it all off. It's quite funny really.

I know that one day, the experience that I have gained will prove useful in my work. Now I think about it, the knowledge that I have gained from this experimentation and creativity has helped me produce music for Claire's meditations and podcasts from this equipment, so whilst it seems there is no great result, actually it has been very useful.

I now have a larger keyboard (MIDI controller) so when the time comes to need more octaves in a composition I can do so. One day I might learn to play the piano properly as well. It's on my bucket list but being honest it's probably a low priority at this point in my life as I have too many other activities and interests to find the time to learn. Until I learn I suppose I just have to continue playing by ear in my way, and that's ok because it can still be enjoyable, creative and useful.

Transformation Key: Some things might have to wait until later and that's ok. It doesn't mean anything good or bad, it just is.

63

17 December 2021: Raging Storms

Raging Storms

There can be seasons within the course of family life that can truly feel like raging storms.

One storm after another can truly test everyone involved.

How we show up during those storms is the true test of character.

As I move along this path of stroke recovery, I learnt pretty damn quickly that family crises shift from one focus to the next in the blink of an eye.

The test of my own character seems difficult x10 due to the impact of brain damage from the stroke. I want to help more. I want to support more. I want to be able to hold my love Claire more in her moments of tears. My own tears flow out of

frustration and anger at the situation(s).
We are human...and sometimes it just feels shit.
But despite the raging storms, my love for my love Claire grows deeper.
I have faith that everything will come good. I have a deeper knowing that at some level all of this madness is for us and not happening to us.
My human easily falls into victim mode but I realise that just perpetuates the trials and challenges. There's no point thinking those thoughts as that will likely attract yet more raging storms. Somewhere there is only light and love. So for this moment, I say thank you Universe; we are learning the lessons (and for me, that's as best as I can in my rather restricted state at present). We focus (as best we can) on the good in everything, whilst moving with grace and forgiveness when we sometimes forget.

As the Winter season of 2021 closed in on Christmas it was accompanied by probably the most difficult period in our family. Claire and I stood together in what felt like a continuous battering of storm after storm. It was a period when our relationship was tested like never before and I felt awful. Awful not because of feeling ill with brain injury but because all I wanted to do was scream and shout at what felt like the injustice of life.

How Claire held it all together is beyond me; I'm not sure that I would have been quite so resilient had it not been for my own recovering state that prevented me from taking more action. I couldn't do anything really, and any form of complexity or problem-solving was completely out of the question for me. If there was a problem to overcome and find a solution for, I'm afraid Claire was predominantly on her own in that period. I am forever indebted to her for holding the fort during that period.

All I could do was do my best to hold her and love her, even though all I wanted was the same back, but to ask or expect that from Claire at that time would have been unreasonable. She needed me as best as I could.

What that meant for me was that I had to dig deeper into my mental reserves more than I had ever been asked to do before. I wasn't sure if I could do it. My human self wanted to say, "What about me? I'm suffering over here too." But I learned to hold that back.

I had the feeling that because my recovery had gone so well up to that point everyone thought I was well again. I have no idea if that's true or not, but it was my overwhelming feeling. I kept thinking to myself, "But I feel crap too, I don't know if I can be the man I'm supposed to be." All I could do was show up with some kind of faith, trust and belief that everything would work out and I promised the universe that I would learn from these lessons.

Transformation Key: When everything seems to be going wrong and things feel like they couldn't get any worse, the truth is they probably could but somehow you will get through it. When you want to give up, don't. You've got this!

64

20 December 2021: Officially Discharged

> *Officially Discharged*
> *...and 14 weeks into stroke recovery I am now officially discharged from the care of my latest Physio Therapy team.*
> *Alice, my physiotherapist, said, "Your improvements are amazing, I can officially discharge you from our care."*
> *Wow, that's some birthday present (birthday tomorrow)*
> *Go me!*

I had mixed feelings when I was discharged from care by the physiotherapy team. Alice was the final physio-therapy nurse assigned to me and she would visit about once every 2 or 3 weeks. She had helped me a lot with both physiotherapy and my mental health as I learnt to comprehend that other family matters were now of higher priority than my recovery from stroke.

When Alice said she was discharging me and wouldn't be coming to see me anymore there was a hint of sadness and a feeling that would now have to deal with all the other family stresses and strains without having her counselling. Now I was alone and I needed to be strong. Claire needed me perhaps more than I needed her (or certainly more than I was prepared to let on). I still wanted to talk things through and seek another perspective on a situation but that was gone for me. Understandably, Claire was distracted by the other family issues that had come into our lives. Alice said she would recommend Psychiatric help for me so that I could talk to someone about my feelings. I was buoyed (mildly) by the fact I would still be able to speak to someone.

On the flip side of being discharged from physiotherapy care, I was over the moon that I had experienced and shown such a strong recovery that physiotherapy (Alice) felt I would be perfectly fit and able to carry on without their care or intervention. That was an incredible achievement at just over 3 months post-stroke. Just 3 months prior I couldn't get out of a hospital bed. Progress had been remarkable!

With my 54th birthday just around the corner, I decided that being discharged from physiotherapy would be an early birthday present.

Transformation Key: It's good to talk. Sometimes all we need is to be heard and that's enough. It is healthy to talk about things that are concerning us. Talking can allow us to hear or see a different perspective on a problem. On other occasions, just the mere act of sharing a problem can help us find relief from that problem.

65

21 December 2021: 54th Birthday

54th Birthday.

Wow, I've made it around the sun another year.

I almost didn't make it when my body had other plans for this year back in September, but hey, here I am.

Did I say how unbelievably grateful I am to be alive? If not, well I am!!!

Claire organised a wonderful day of celebration and I am so blessed in every possible way!

She had arranged that all the younger children came over (our Bryony is a long way away in Australia) and then we all, along with Claire's mum and dad Roger and Anita and Toby the dog, went to Ogmore by Sea.

It was cold but to be outside at the coast felt amazing today.

It felt so incredibly good to be alive!!! Happy happy happy happy Thank you Claire for everything you do. Words cannot describe how perfect and spot-on you make everything! You're amazing.

So Happy Birthday to me and everyone I know who shares this special birthday.

Also, Happy Winter Solstice to all. It's a magical time when we can celebrate all things winter and look forward to the springtime that will start to unfold before us (my favourite time of year).

Also, for any Rush fans, Happy 2112 day!! Classic album!!

...and finally for anyone in the entertainment industry, Happy microphone testing day, 211221...stupid I know, but hey.

Feeling amazing

Happy 54th!! Blimey, I almost didn't make it at all. That's a sobering thought. But if I wasn't supposed to make then I wouldn't have I suppose. Having such a close call with death certainly does make one look at life differently, or perhaps I should say in several different ways. There's an undeniable greater sense of gratitude for one's life. The fact that being alive in the first place is an absolute miracle and against the odds. Then there's the feeling of ok, if it is my time to die then don't sweat it. Who am I to resist the will of God? If it's my time then it's my time. Yes, that's shit but if my time is up, well my time is up.

When Claire said we were heading to Ogmore-by-sea for my

birthday, I was pleased. "Oggy" is one of my favourite places to see some coastline. It takes about 1.5 hours to drive there, but it's worth the drive in my opinion. When we went for my birthday it was cold and bleak which is typical for my birthday. The 21st of December is the Winter solstice in the Northern Hemisphere (aka the shortest day of the year, aka the least amount of sunlight). I celebrate the day not only because of my birthday but also because it signifies a change and turning point in the seasonal cycle. The long dark days of the winter months are changing and the light from the sun will be extending as we head towards spring and summer. Yes!!

Throughout my life, I've always had a dislike for winter and the darker days. That was until I met Claire. She has made winter and my birthday very special. She has treated me to some incredible short holidays and breaks abroad for my birthday. This year was obviously going to be different because of my stroke recovery and then we had the added turmoil with family matters and then we also didn't have a clue where any money was going to be coming from, In previous years we had been away to various places like Corfe Castle near Swanage in Dorset, Edinburgh and even Rome for my 50th birthday where we also got engaged. Thanks to Claire, wintertime and my birthday have become a time of celebration, perhaps in the way that they always should have been.

This year we went to Ogmore-by-sea to celebrate with all the family with plenty of cold sea air. It was a great day as we visited the beach and the small castle and walked along a small stretch of coastline before the cold got the better of us.

It was family life at its best and it gave everyone a moment of relief from the madness of that year.

Transformation Key: Sometimes just do what you can. It doesn't have to be some grand gesture or make a big statement. Just make it intentional as that is enough.

66

✸

22 December 2021: Den Building

Den building

Having fun in the woods building dens with the kids and friends.

Stroke survival recovery continues with this fun exercise. It was cold but we were determined to try to build something.

Unfortunately, we ran out of long solid sticks so we had to abandon our efforts and take the dog for his walk.

Our amazing friends Gemma and Kevin and their son Jack were incredible supporters to our entire family as we navigated the rough waves on a metaphorical ocean that seemed destined to destroy us.

Gemma and Kevin helped Claire in the initial days when I was hospitalised in Oxford. Without any hesitation or question, they took hold of Claire and transported her to and from Oxford and made sure she was fed and supplied with coffee and chia lattes when Claire couldn't think or fend for herself. Gemma also provided Claire with a much-needed shoulder to cry on and lots of hugs after visiting me in the Oxford hospital.

After my discharge from Swindon Hospital Gemma would pop over with meals and both Gemma and Kevin were able to give direct support to the kids when they needed to talk to someone outside of the immediate family. In short Gemma and Kevin are amazing people that are truly loved by our entire family.

The woods provide my family and I with one of the best playgrounds and of course in fitting with the woodland setting is the opportunity to build dens.

Den building is a great activity for us all, but on this particular day, I was pleased to be involved and get my brain working differently. We had to work together to design a shelter or den.

Gemma and Jack joined in even though it wasn't a very nice day. I think it might have been a bit cold for them both and the lack of good den-building sticks made the process rather tough going for us all. We had to eventually concede defeat and give up our den-building adventures for the day. That said, I did enjoy the experience and it was great (as always) to be out in the cold fresh air.

We returned home to the warmth and freshly made cup of tea and festive mince pie (of course). Was life finally returning to some form of normality? No, but these small moments of joy, it was a chance to forget all the hardships and just enjoy the 'now' moment of trying to build a den in the woods.

Transformation Key: Grab each opportunity to live whenever the moment arises. Live for 'now' and don't wait for circumstances to change.

67

23 December 2021: Festive Joy

> *Festive Joy*
>
> *... it is my absolute pleasure to be able to wish all my friends here on FB the very best of joy for this festive season.*
>
> *As many know, our family and I have been through tests and trials in these past few months, but through love, we know we will be stronger than ever...and it is from the perspective of a "full cup" of love that we extend our love and joy to all our friends, family and connections in this season of joy and celebration.*
>
> *May love, joy and happiness be yours in abundance now and forever.*

I don't suppose it crossed my mind until the moment I posted this message on 23 Dec 2021, but I was incredibly lucky to have even reached the point of sending Christmas wishes to anyone. When I stopped to think about it, had the cards fallen differently, I could have been dead and this would be Christmas without Simon, without Dad! Phew, even writing this brings up tears and emotions. Sadness, coupled with the joy of being alive. Very mixed emotions.

The secret to finding such peace in the festive season and in the moment was the absolute deepest recognition of the abundance of love.

Transformation Key: Love is the light that will illuminate the way in the darkest of seasons.

68

24 December 2021:
Christmas Scare

Christmas Scare

Yesterday I started slurring my speech.

I went to bed, and had a good night's sleep, but woke up this morning still slurring.

I have to admit, I was concerned but I felt fine except for the speech. I didn't want to spend hours in A&E... not today, not on Christmas Eve. If there was some way to have a CT Scan then please let that happen. I needed to understand what was going on but not by the A&E route.... Please no!!!

An ambulance arrived on the doorstep like a miracle and the crew checked me out and said that I should go to hospital but given my recent history, they would recommend to admissions that I go straight in for a CT Scan.

> *So, I was blue-lighted to hospital. The tears flowed as I thought the worst....no not again!!! I was fully conscious and very aware of the speed we were going. I could hear the sirens. We were moving fast!! That made me cry even more.*
>
> *Kris from the ambulance crew held my hand reassuring me that everything would be ok. He was my guardian angel this morning. He called ahead insisting that I go straight into CT....omg he was brilliant.*
>
> *The CT Scan has shown no bleeds at all and the neurology consultant is happy with my condition....*
> *...I'm going home for Christmas*

Miracles can happen! Really! So here I was on Christmas Eve of 2021 and I needed a real Christmas miracle. In the days leading up to Christmas, I had started to feel 'off'. I was getting stressed out because it looked like both of my parents were going to spend their Christmases in the hospital. Neither of them were well enough to be at home and that made me sad. I wanted to send them both a small gift so that they would be able to open something from me and the family whilst in the hospital.

Because of the uncertainty surrounding whether Mum or Dad were going to be at their respective homes for Christmas, it was becoming increasingly unlikely that I would be able to get anything mailed out to them to arrive in time for Christmas Day. Also, my brain couldn't think straight to ask the right questions of anyone to help me fathom a solution to the problem. I remember that I decided to buy a magazine each that they would enjoy.

On Dec 23, I drove into the local town with Charlotte for company. I suppose I took someone with me to help me and Charlotte did do her best, bless her.

We found the magazines I wanted to send and we figured out appropriate sturdy envelopes to mail them in. We returned home to write the addresses as Mum and Dad were in two separate hospitals, Gloucester Royal and Swindon GWH.

Having found the addresses, wrote the envelopes, and packed the magazines, I then set off back into town before the post office shut for Christmas. This time our two boys wanted to come with me (William and Logan). For them, this was just a trip into town.

We parked the van in the high street and marched to the post office, mindful that time was slipping away and the post office would be closing anytime soon.

We made it. We stood in the queue waiting our turn.

I had a mask over my nose and mouth due to the masking rules of the pandemic. The post office worker behind the counter looked at me and I tried to speak...

I couldn't speak properly.

I initially thought it was the mask causing the speech

difficulty. I persevered and I managed to pay for the packages to be posted and then left with the boys in tow. Job done!

We returned to the van and having climbed in I remember looking at my mouth in the rearview mirror. I was checking to see if my face looked weird. Had my face dropped to one side? I couldn't feel it properly. It felt numb. It felt like I had been injected with an anaesthetic to numb any pain in the dentist. But of course, I hadn't. This was weird.

Also in these few days, between my birthday and leading up to Christmas, I noticed that my blood pressure had been increasing. My reading on Dec 23, 2021, was 140/101 which is high. The diastolic reading of 101 was not good news.

Shit, was a having another stroke? Oh no, what was happening?

I returned home with the boys and I rested up for the remainder of the day in the hope that good sleep would help restore my speech and everything would be all right in the morning of Christmas Eve (Dec 24, 2021).

I awoke on Christmas Eve and went to the bathroom. I checked my face in the mirror and tried to speak to myself in the mirror. The speech was still impaired and the numb feeling in one side of my mouth was still apparent. I felt utterly deflated. All the good progress I had been making was just gone!

Claire asked me what I wanted to do. "I don't know!" I said

in despair. "I don't want to spend hours (all day) in the A&E department at the hospital on Christmas Eve, no way!" I thought to myself. I couldn't articulate that very well and so Claire was having a hard time understanding me. Charlotte could hear the concern in Claire's voice and appeared in the bedroom. "What's going on with Dad ?" she asked in a very concerned way. Claire explained as best she could.

To my astonishment, Charlotte had messaged her Mum (my ex-wife Jo) about my problem.

As Claire and I were discussing what to do without getting to any conclusion, I heard one of the children shout up the stairs, "There's an ambulance outside."

I heard Claire go downstairs to speak to one of the paramedics. I heard a conversation that went something like this:

Claire, "We haven't called an ambulance."

Paramedic, "We've been called out to this address, is there anyone that needs our help?"

Claire, " Well actually, I have a concern with my partner. He's upstairs"

Paramedic, "Do you mind if we come in and take a look at him?"

Claire, "No, not at all, please come in."

Two paramedics entered the bedroom and took over.

The one who spoke with me was called Kris. A beautiful co-incidence that I should get Kris on Christmas Eve.

Claire also spoke with Kris explaining my stroke history and between the three of us we managed to convey my concern about being funnelled straight into A&E so Kris said, "We'll get you straight in for a CT Scan." Kris was not messing about. I don't think he wanted a stroke death on his Christmas Eve shift. He promised me that he would call ahead en route to the hospital and get us straight into the CT Scanner. With that promise, I agreed to go.

Here we go again, another blue light trip in the back of an ambulance. But this time I was conscious. Unlike the previous two times, I had been blue-lighted in the back of an ambulance, I could hear and sense everything that was happening. On the previous occasions, I had been unconscious and I was convinced that it wasn't possible to hear the sirens whilst in the back of an ambulance. "How very wrong am I!?", I thought. I could hear the sirens easily. The thought of spending Christmas in the hospital upset me. The thought of having a major setback upset me. The thought of having another stroke and medical complications upset me. I wept as we travelled at high speed. Kris held my hand to offer an essential human touch in that desperate time of need.

As he had promised, Kris radioed ahead to get clearance to head straight to the CT Scanning area of Swindon GWH. We arrived and sure enough, there was no hanging around in A&E, it was straight in for a CT Scan for me!

Lo and behold, there I was waiting for a minute or two while they opened up the CT Scan area. I was told by Kris that this was the brand new CT Scanner for Swindon Hospital, totally state-of-the-art technology!

In I went. Kris bid me fair well and good luck.

I had the CT Scan and was then wheeled on a stretcher into an area called Resus to await the results, I was in bay Resus 3 as I recall.

As I lay there, the nurse who was with me was the very same nurse who had seen me on the day of the haemorrhage, some 3 months earlier. Her name was Amy. Claire had spoken to me about Amy and how brilliant she was but this was the first time I could remember meeting Amy.

She greeted me warmly like an old friend. When I think about it, being greeted warmly by a senior stroke nurse is not an ideal situation to be fair! Anyway, it was nice to be with someone who recognised and knew me I suppose. We chatted about her work shift over the upcoming Christmas period while we waited for the results.

The results came in.

Amy casually said, "Everything looks fine, no further bleeding."

This was music to my ears!

"So I can go home then?" I asked expectantly.

"Yes, there is no need to be here. The consultant will come through and explain everything in a moment", Amy replied.

The consultant appeared and stood at the end of the hospital bed on which I was lying. In his strong East European accent, he started to explain but I didn't understand a word of it. All I knew was that there was no further bleeding in my brain and I could go home.

It really did feel like Christmas and miracles do happen!

Amy said I could call Claire to come and get me and that the entire episode was probably due to stress.

"Go home and rest, and enjoy your Christmas", she said.

I think I cried tears of joy.

Transformation Key: Miracles do happen. The best thing you can do is just get out of the way to let the universe do its thing.

69

25 December 2021:
Christmas 2021 in
Recovery

Christmas 2021 in Recovery

These last few days have been very hard. I cannot begin to express how grateful I am to have been home for Christmas and I am so appreciative to all my family especially Claire and her parents for the incredible hard work that it takes to make Christmas special for everyone. I could not do anything towards it this year; they have made it special despite so many hardships right now. Thank you guys!!

On the 23rd Dec, my speech started to slur, I've also noticed my balance had got a lot worse. My recovery took a big step backwards.

This has made me very sad. My human is pissed off and yet I know from the CT scan I had yesterday that I've not had any re-bleed in my brain (thank God)so in that sense this is just a setback on my recovery journey.

Nonetheless, it's hard to take this setback. I've got no choice but to release all control and let go.

This is so hard for me. I feel very lonely inside my body, I wanted to say "broken" body then, but I resisted. I don't say I'm broken.

I still recognise that I'm a survivor and not a victim, but some days I really do want to play the victim card... I am pissed off; I hate this situation; I want to scream and shout; I had to take a moment today to just cry I've done quite a lot of that in these last 2 days.

Sometimes I feel like a burden to Claire, I know she's exhausted with so many life challenges from every direction at the moment, so I don't help with my own recovery challenges. I find it so frustrating that I cannot help her and worse still, I think the truth is I probably add to her woes!

Tomorrow I'll go for another day, digging deep to restart and build my recovery again.

There are small dark moments when I want to give up but the overwhelming urge is to keep going so that I can get to the other side of this shit storm and truly learn the lessons so I can pass them on to others.

I know there are deep learnings somewhere in all this madness. Here's to a new day

It was hard in those days leading up to Christmas. There was so much going "wrong" in our family that it became very close to being too much to bear for me. It was probably one of the toughest times of our lives and I felt so completely helpless and afraid. What was remarkable was that Claire and I remained strong in our love for one another. We faced so much that seemed to come at us. It was like being tossed around in a tint boat in a raging sea. I can imagine wave after wave battering our tiny boat with our family clinging on for life whilst the waves seemed to get bigger and bigger.

I'm not sure how the relationship between Claire and I survived that period but it did; we did; and we grew stronger as a result. I have no desire to go there again as it was so deeply tested.

In terms of my recovery, it took a battering too, but the news that I hadn't had a re-bleed in my brain seemed to carry me along and helped me navigate the difficulties.

Due to my injured brain, I could only surrender to the circumstances. I had no other choice. Perhaps my injured brain did me a favour. Because I had no choice but to surrender to the circumstances and take whatever was coming to me, it somehow allowed a greater level of resilience.

As I write this now looking back on that time I still don't quite know how I navigated it all. That said, I suppose the greatest learning from that time was that no matter how desperate the situation, Claire and I remained strong and together, and that the love of family can hold everything together. The learning is that great love is unshakeable even when tested by circumstances that are beyond our control. As they say, "Love conquers all."

Transformation Key: Love is the guiding light that can hold everything together.

70

26 December 2021: My Human Wants To Cry

My Human wants to cry
...and yet my soul wants to sing for being alive!
I live in both perspectives simultaneously.
Is it hard? Absolutely!
I want this sh!t to stop but I'll continue this journey as best I can....navigating the madness and always looking for the beauty.

I thought that the period leading up to Christmas was bad, but between Christmas and New Year, I fell into a deep feeling of depression with regular bouts of suicidal ideation.

It was a time of deep torment for my soul. I felt so utterly beaten and defeated and yet so deeply grateful for being alive with the good news that I had received on Christmas Eve. I felt guilty for feeling so bad, which made things worse. It was such a profound juxtaposition of emotions simultaneously flying through my body. I felt so alone, and I felt that no one would be able to get through to me had they tried. I wasn't sure that I even wanted anyone to get through. I still don't know whether Claire and her family knew how desperate I felt. I suppose they must have known something was deeply wrong, but I couldn't articulate how desperate I felt.

I had a heavy cold. I wasn't sure if I had picked up COVID-19 or not, but dared not take an LFT test for fear that it would inflict yet more bad news upon my already battered soul and nervous system. Deep inside I knew that what I had picked up was a heavy winter cold, and that was all, but I still kept myself in self-isolation to be sure. To be honest, it suited me to be in self-isolation at that time anyway. Mentally, I was completely done; finished. My mental health hit rock bottom and I had to find myself again before re-surfacing and interacting with the family. I couldn't put on the brave face and smile anymore, I was completely drained of any positivity.

This dark period lasted until New Year's Day.

Transformation Key: With every breakdown a breakthrough can bloom.

71

26 December 2021:
Precious Moments

Precious Moments

I can't lie. Navigating life is f..king hard at the moment but it's times like these that make it worth living for!

Today, we picked up my youngest kids having dropped off Claire's kids (all change).

We decided to just completely chill out - Claire and I needed that more than ever. I feel so sorry for Claire at the moment.

We spent time walking in the fresh air with the dog. It was lovely to be out although I could only manage a short distance before we returned home to grab some lovely Christmas dinner leftovers and then chilled in front of the TV and films.

Ok, heading to bed now as I've also caught a heavy cold - great, not!!

Despite feeling utterly defeated by life I still had to make the effort with my kids. We hadn't been with them on Christmas Day and they came over to us the following day, Boxing Day here in the UK.

We went out for a walk and some cold fresh winter air. Fresh air always re-energises. We returned home to enjoy some left-over Christmas dinner and then watched some films together.

Generally, I'm not one for vegging out and chilling in front of the TV, but getting lost in a good film can be fun, especially with the kids.

Transformation Key: Sometimes making the effort to do something can make a difference and can re-energise you; try it!

72

⁘

27 December 2021: Surrounded By Love Yet Feeling So Lonely

Surrounded by love yet feeling so lonely.

I know what I want to say but my mouth won't form the words. This inability to communicate orally creates a feeling of great loneliness. I feel kind of trapped in my own body... I can only imagine the horror of locked-in syndrome!!! Argh, that must be awful!!

I know that I am surrounded by the love of my family and when they take the piss out of me it's actually easier for me ...some of the kids call me "specy" cos I'm now "special" or have "special needs". To be the object of their humour is actually ok, I can laugh with them. I've always had the ability to laugh at myself.... I'm so grateful for that gift right now.

But sometimes when the communication is difficult I just want to retreat and withdraw; it's easier. It's easier than having to try the communication again, the moment has gone, the humour in the split second has passed, people don't get it, they can't hear me. It's not their fault.

I mumble like an incoherent fool. My words don't make sense.

Toothpaste Is now thoothpaze

Coffee please is now Othee peez

I mean FFS my loved ones don't have a chance, do they??! And I sit there in the middle of this BS trying to be normal. I can't be normal; I'm not normal at this time; what does normal even mean anyway? I think it will start with being able to communicate again effectively.

14 weeks ago I was knocked off my feet...my ability to balance was taken from me.

4 days ago my ability to communicate was taken from me....

So no more setbacks please universe. I know you're listening so I'd now like:

Peace

Health

Money

I would like to feel safe and secure again, please. No more scary shit ok?

I'm still alive so I'm grateful for that ....

One day this will all make sense I'm sure....

In the meantime, I'll just learn to perfect screaming inside....and

continue to breathe deeply.
....argh....

Oh my goodness this was a very tough time. I wanted to scream inside and curl up and die. Why? Why? Why? I was not a happy man. But something kept me going... humour maybe?

Eva, one of our middle daughters, Claire's eldest child, started to refer to me (well everyone) as 'Specky' about being in special need (nice one Eva). Anyway, it seemed quite fitting and it became a thing in the house. One might frown upon such a name, but as I was the subject of the name (along with others), I approved of it and played along with the joke; it made me smile and laugh. I was desperate for any form of lightheartedness in that period so if being called "Specky" provided that relief then that was fine by me.

Transformation Key: Humour is fantastic medicine, alleviating mental, emotional and physical dis-ease. Try to find something to lift the mood a little and laugh. Maybe a funny film or podcast might help. Suffering can ease with laughter.

73

28 December 2021: Time To Mend

Time to mend.

I need time to mend, to heal my broken body. I thought I was progressing well but then the time between my birthday and Christmas 2021 dealt me a blow and a setback I was not expecting.

Claire has been amazing. She is giving me the space to rest and heal. I think without that space, I would tip over the edge in a bigger and badder way (yep I made up the word).

I'm reading a book that my brother got me for my birthday called The Salt Path... a redemptive story of a couple who had lost everything but then found everything walking the Salt Path of the southwest coast of England.

The story reminds me of the trip Claire and I took to South

> *Wales last August 2021. I recall the sheer cliffs and danger. Some of the visions of looming cliffs bearing down on us are etched in my mind so clearly. Were these cliffs foreboding the most testing time of our lives....who knows, maybe. Were they warning of danger ahead?*
>
> *For now, my job is to mend, to grow stronger again and one day I'll become the new man I am supposed to be. I'll find him again soon, I'm sure. and when I do we'll walk those same cliffs again. I love you, Claire*

Reading the book "The Salt Path" during the time around Christmas and New Year might not have helped my nervous system to be honest. The true story is amazing but I couldn't help drawing close comparisons to the poor desperate people in the story and the plight that Claire and I were facing.

I didn't know where our income was coming from. It was one of the scariest times in my life; I felt the pressure bearing down on me but of course, I was not capable of anything. All my abilities to work in my former capacity were stripped from me. I had no one calling me about contracts. Nothing! I would lie in my bed at night wondering how we were going to keep our house. The story that I was reading was about how a couple had lost their home and their former life following some terrible misfortunes and one of them faced a crippling illness that would threaten to eventually take his body and end his life. I won't spoil the book for anyone else but it is really gripping and I thoroughly recommend it.

Claire and I were not at that level of desperation (we still had our house), but in my mind, it was hell. To add to the fear about money and our finances that welled up in my body and mind, it was desperately cold weather. I would read about how the couple walking the Salt Path would camp out and have to cope with the wind and rain on England's South Western coastline. I could picture dangerous cliffs and rugged drops into the sea from the descriptions in the story and my memories of visits to the coastline of South West England and Wales.

One such visit was in August 2021 just before the stroke. We stayed in a beautiful wooden yurt close to a stretch of coastline in South Wales on the Bristol Channel between Llanwit Major and Ogmore by sea. It has stunning cliffs but they are very dangerous and appear threatening with their great heights.

The only way you can pass below the cliffs is to walk between specific points at low tide. You have to monitor the tide times very carefully because the tide in that area can rise by something like 7m. I recall being told that it was the second highest in terms of low tide vs. high tide in the world. It's not a place you want to get caught by the incoming tide as there is no means of escape! It's just the sea and huge dangerous cliffs.

I remember Claire and I walked a stretch of low-tide beach near Nash Point Lighthouse to Monknash Beach. We had looked up the tides to ensure we could make it, but it was still pretty scary. For the majority of the walk, all we could see was a rocky beach, massive looming cliffs, a rising sea getting ever closer and farther ahead a headland that looked difficult to walk around. There was no way off this stretch of coast. We had never walked it before and we didn't have a map or Google Maps to tell us where we would find the point we had been told about earlier where we could get off the beach to safety. We either had to keep going without being able to see the escape route or quit and turn back quickly to beat the rising tide. We marched pretty bloody quickly keeping faith that we could get around the headland as we had been told earlier and it would reveal our means of escape from the beach.

We kept going and made it to safety with just minutes to go before the tide would have blocked our way. We had made it. Thank God! That night I remember having a nightmare waking up at about 2 a.m. so fearful of the looming cliffs we had seen that day.

In the period around Christmas and New Year, facing the threat of financial ruin (as I thought), feeling utterly defeated and depressed and reading the story of a couple having lost everything sleeping in a tent on the coast, I was facing all those demons again. It was horrible. But this time I could not do anything about it. I had no choice but to surrender! We both had to rely on whatever income Claire could generate which was good but very sporadic and of course, she was focused in almost every different direction with juggling the family, Christmas, homeschooling, supporting me and her business...and all I could do was focus on my recovery. For me, as someone who had taken on the provider role (rightly or wrongly), it was intensely worrying and frustrating, but I also knew that I had to focus on myself, and my well-being and somehow find the inner strength to work through my fears and demons.

Transformation Key: Even though your ego-mind might be screaming at you and filling you with worry and fear, there will come a point where the only thing to do is surrender. That doesn't mean quitting. It means surrender to the unknown. Surrender control of having everything worked out. Sometimes you have to trust and believe that the universe does have your back!

74

〆⊗

29 December 2021: Blood Pressure

Blood Pressure

I have written on a number of occasions about how my brain haemorrhage (stroke) was caused by high blood pressure/ hypertension.

I monitor my blood pressure (almost daily) and I now take meds to help bring it down along with other lifestyle changes.

Over the Christmas period, I caught a heavy cold and I've noticed the effect on my increased BP.

I've avoided regular cold remedies as they are known to increase BP but still, it's interesting to observe that one of the body responses to a heavy cold seems to be increased BP. I didn't know that.

So, I'm not going to freak out over it. I'll still take my meds,

> *I'll still do my yoga hopefully without falling over), and I'll continue to walk the dog in the fresh air and nature....all good relievers of stress....I'll just do it all gently.*
> *What's the lesson? Being kind to myself and not let things (eg. increasing BP) mean anything.*
> *Have a great day*

When I learnt to be kind to myself, I realised just how much power that could give me.

It's a phrase that I had first heard used about 6 or 7 years earlier but I realised I had never really understood it. In late 2014, I found myself in another difficult set of circumstances, I had lost my job, I had lost my marriage and I had lost my home. A kind lady from my place of work in the US Headquarters had said to me "Be kind to yourself" as we wished each other farewell on the day I left my job. At the time I just thanked her and didn't think much more of it. That was until late 2021.

That late 2021 period had brought up all manner of reasons to be kind to myself. Life had given me a good kick. I was completely depleted of all my energy. Somehow I had survived a brain haemorrhage almost 4 months earlier, but here I was in a complete mess. Life had dealt me a pile of shit and somehow there would be a way through, but that way through had yet to reveal itself, or perhaps there was no way through at all and maybe it would have been better if I had died! This was the sort of rubbish flying through my head at the time.

Sometimes, I just wanted to throw all my toys out of the pram and hold myself a big old pity party. But something kept me going. Something enabled me to find another deeper level of mental strength to hold on to. The phrase of being kind to myself re-entered my head from 7 years previous. Perhaps that was the thing that kept me going. The concept of really, truly, deeply being kind to myself might have been enough to help me hold onto a vision of a better outcome even though my present reality was anything like the vision I still trusted would come to pass, eventually.

Each day in that period I measured my blood pressure. I suppose it was a precautionary strategy on my part because I was so stressed out I didn't want another bleed to occur.

I noticed that it had risen slightly and was now back in the high blood pressure range, although thankfully, nothing like 4 months earlier when I'd had the brain haemorrhage.

Despite the rise in blood pressure I decided to not sweat about it. Worrying about that would most likely make it worse. You are what you think, so if I thought and worried about having high blood pressure, that is exactly what I would create, high blood pressure. On the outside, I blamed the increase in BP on my heavy cold (which may well have been a contributing factor) but I think it was a combination of stress factors on my body. Whatever the cause, I decided the best course of action was to be kind to myself and allow myself peace to allow myself to create better health and mental well-being for myself.

Transformation Key: Be kind to yourself. By finding a space of peace, we can also find an ability to be kind to ourselves to allow deeper healing to occur.

75

29 December 2021: Walking Again

Walking again.

Slowly but surely I'm finding the mental and physical strength to start walking outside again.

I must admit that having a heavy cold on top of the setback that happened on the 23rd and 24th Dec has really messed me up mentally.

I've had numerous suicidal thoughts (that I dismissed swiftly) and the mental pain of this period has been harder than ever.

Yesterday and today I walked out with Toby. Sometimes I stopped to cry or take a picture or two. This whole Christmas period has been far from easy. I think Christmas is difficult for a lot of people so I know I'm not alone.

Roll on springtime (my favourite time of year) but in the

> *meantime, I'll feel the emotion of the unhealed pain trapped in my body.*
>
> *I'll work through the sadness that has been in there for years. Probably 7 years or more. I'll cry the tears because I know the release will be forever. Once the sadness is out it's out and if there's any remaining I'll cry some more until the tears turn to laughter which they always do.*
>
> *Here's to walking again; here's to healing inside and out. Here's to healing permanently and finding joy on the other side.*

It was during the period between Christmas and New Year that my truest healing began. This was the emotional healing from past trauma that had stayed in my body for years.

It was a period when suicidal ideation reared its ugly head once more. I would be walking towards the woods and a flash of suicidal thought would punctuate my thoughts almost as if my mind were reaching for some relief from the deepest depression that I felt I was in. Almost instantaneously, as soon as the suicidal thought had appeared, it would be replaced by another thought of guilt and an image of my kids and Claire in tears. "How could I do that to them?" I thought to myself, and that was quickly followed by, "I can't do that to them, no way." So somehow this internal conversation would float away until the next time.

As I walked, I relished the joy of being outside again. I relished the joy and beauty of nature, and in that glimmer of joy I found a reason to keep going, a deep determination but I knew I had healing to do.

"So let the healing commence", I thought to myself. The depth of my despair in that period allowed me to reach places within me where hurt and pain had been covered up by my ego mind to protect me from feeling that trauma once again. "Thanks for your help ego-mind, but I've got this now. I have to face this hurt and pain once more so that I can finally let it go."

To be finally free from years and years of emotional trauma I had to feel it all again. I cried and cried, and as I cried the weight in my heart lifted. Inexplicable, the tears would turn to laughter without any rationale. My mind could not apply a logical reason for the tears, but that was the whole point, my rational mind, in its attempt to protect me from further pain, had pushed the emotional hurt and pain deeper inside my body. The healing was underway. What a relief.

Transformation Key: It's good to cry. Holding onto emotional pain and trauma can be extremely unhealthy.

76

30 December 2021: Surrendering

Surrendering

For me, this does not mean giving up or rolling over with my legs in the air like a dying fly.

No, I've come to re-realise (ie. Realise again and again) that surrendering means submitting to God's will.

I love it when I speak with friends of different faiths. Why? Because no matter what the faith there is a universal acceptance of a God (higher power / higher intelligence) that spans all faiths. This is the God I refer to. This is the God I want to connect with more. This is the God that I surrender to.

I always had a belief in this universal God...and I choose to call it God because that's nice and short and easy. There are all manner of names but I choose God.

As a 7-year-old child, I recall being asked to draw God in a school class. I drew a power station. Why not? That is my God....pure source energy and infinite intelligence...beyond words, beyond description or logic.

Some might call this my "come to Jesus moment"

The truth is I came to Jesus long long ago, Jesus, Allah, Buddha, they're all wise messengers in my world. Even a f...king power station when I was 7 years old. There are no rules, no limits in my world. No judgement, only just what is....and it's all ok.Back to surrender...

Perhaps the truth is I didn't really surrender in the past. I thought all this stuff but always held back for fear of judgement from others. Probably. I protected my ego. I didn't want conflict or invite a disagreement. I lived in fear.

I believe with absolute faith that there has to be some meaning in all this. I know that the meaning will be revealed one day, in some way. It will all make sense. I'm confident that the truth will be shown as I surrender. Surrendering at this point means speaking my absolute truth no matter what fears are presented.

I trust. I believe. All will be revealed.

Have a blessed day

Surrendering to God's will is surrendering or accepting that maybe there is a divine plan that I am a part of but I am not an orchestrator of. My ego-mind has found that idea hard to accept for most of my life but maybe I was wrong all that time.

There is so much in our world that cannot be explained by science. I've always had a deeper knowing that there is something far bigger than ourselves at play but words cannot describe that knowing, it just is.

When I drew a power station in my school class as a 7-year-old boy, I knew then deep in my heart that I had a knowing that could not be explained. Why would a country boy who had never seen a power station decide to draw one as a representation of God at 7 years old? I still don't know to this day, what made me draw that power station but perhaps it was my higher self (the God within me) trying to speak to me/us to express the unlimited source of power that lies within each of us. That power is universal and spans all religions and faiths, all colours and creeds, all species, every plant, every tree, every living and formerly living thing and everything in our universe, and so it is that that power resides in all of us; it's universal and it's everywhere and I understood that when I was 7.

It is this power that I chose to surrender to. I had faith and knew that pushing against this power was a futile exercise. To resist that power would cause yet more harm to my body. The power of God wanted to get through. The time had come to embrace God in my heart again. I didn't know what would happen. Would the clouds part and God (the power station) appear from the sky? I had no idea and I had no expectation of anything, I just knew it was time.

Transformation Key: There may come a point when God/the Universe/Divine Intelligence/Source Energy speaks to your heart. Let that knowing soothe your tired heart, let that knowing replenish your body. Let that knowing be your power and your fuel.

77

31 December 2021: Exercise Routine

Exercise routine.
Walking through the woods, through the mud, slipping on the wet roots...and then avoiding the low branches.
This is all good physiotherapy for a stroke survivor.

For someone recovering from stroke and traumatic brain injury, the act of walking around the woodland in the wintertime provides a fantastic exercise and physiotherapy routine.

The slippery roots and branches are pretty lethal for anyone, let alone someone who feels constantly drunk and dizzy. But it is that danger that makes it all the more challenging I suppose.

Mud is another major hazard and my boots leaked! They didn't have huge holes in but somewhere they leaked in moisture (mmm, no let's say water, and muddy water at that). So I would try to avoid walking in the wet, squelchy mud because of the risk of leakage through to my socks, but the foul, wet mud was always present at that time of year and it was very slippery.

So underfoot it was fairly hazardous, but to add to the danger were the low branches from fallen trees or trees that had decided that it was a good idea to grow in a sideways direction rather than an upward direction (it's all about reaching the sunlight I suppose). There is one particular area that provided great physiotherapy in the form of mud, roots and very low-level branches. I would gingerly make my way through this particular obstacle and then duck back and forth under the lower, fallen branches, pausing after each duck to feel the increased dizziness in my head, before letting it settle and then repeating the exercise. On a good day, it wouldn't be raining when I did this. Unfortunately, it was seldom sunny in the middle of winter.

Transformation Key: The brain needs to be tested and pushed to make new neurological pathways and new neurology is the basis of all transformation.

78

1 January 2022: Peace In Uncertainty

Peace in Uncertainty.

Moving forward in 2022.

How do you deal with intense uncertainty?

With Grace, with forgiveness, with courage, with hope

It is with these qualities that we are able to:

Move forward without having the benefit of foresight

We move forward without having the benefit of clear plans

We move forward without having the benefit of safety

We move forward without having the benefit of clarity

To have certainty provides our human a sense of safety. Certainty brings comfort and well-being.

But for those of us without that certainty, and there are many of us, we can find peace in the unknown.

For it is in the unknown, that place of pure potentiality, that we will find our truth and our greatest healing. Beyond the wall of comfort lies a greater love than we can ever know.

Whilst we remain in the comfort (zone) there is no growth, there is no expansion.

And as much as this uncertainty (as we enter this bright New Year of 2022) can limit our vision, it can limit our sense of destiny. It is through Grace Forgiveness Courage and Hope that we can move forward, embracing the uncertain, embracing the unknown, in such a way that we see it as incredible possibilities and opportunities for salvation.

The fear of the unknown can easily bring us to a standstill. We can be held fast by our fears. When we choose to let our fears determine the next step, we do not move forward, we do not progress, we do not expand, we do not grow.

So whilst we embrace this exciting New Year, there will be (with certainty) an increasing level of uncertainty, which we must embrace and overcome so we can live our best year ever.

In 2021, I learned that nothing in life is certain. I am not alone. So many had life-changing events thrust upon them. No certainty. Complete disruption. But with Grace, Courage, Forgiveness and Hope we can see a way through to the love and peace on the other side.

With all my love

Happy New Year 2022

Uncertainty is one of the four nouns that make up the

acronym VUCA (volatility, uncertainty, complexity and ambiguity). VUCA is a term originated by the US military but used in other fields to represent the situation often seen with or associated with intense change.

Almost everything in my life seemed uncertain in those first days of 2022, but through faith and belief and an ability to muster grace, forgiveness, courage and hope, I managed to navigate my way through the fog of uncertainty.

With grace and forgiveness coupled with courage and hope, I found a sense of peace despite the intense uncertainty.

Grace and Forgiveness worked as a pair as did Courage and Hope. I would forgive myself for being scared and in that forgiveness I found a grace for myself that soothed my soul. Through my faith and belief, I found that my hope for the future increased and that fuelled my courage.

Some might say that faith is blind faith and in a way that is exactly what having faith is. It is blind faith. The nature of true faith is blind. It's an ability to believe and trust even though there is no evidence to support that belief. Some might say that having blind faith is foolhardy but when all options were fading away, sometimes blind faith was all I had left. The secret to faith is becoming completely okay with blind faith. Faith, trust and belief transcend into a form of knowing. I started to know (don't ask me how) that everything would work out ok.

Transformation Key: Having true faith is having blind faith.

There will be many who will oppose your faith by attempting to aggravate fears and doubts within you.

79

5 January 2021: Reboot

Reboot

There's a thing about Stoke that is more striking than anything else, and that is that life will never be the same again!

This can be both good and bad, and which perspective I choose can flip from one to the other in a moment.

The thing is though, the choice is mine.

I have to be honest, some days it's hard. I miss the person I was. You lose yourself as a result of Stroke....and for that, some days I hate this f...king Stroke! It's almost impossible to describe that feeling to anyone else. To others on the outside, I may look "normal", but on the inside, I feel anything but "normal". Endless brain fog is so frustrating. The ability to process data is hard...especially if half the data is missing! I need data in exact clarity in order to try to make sense of a situation...the normal healthy human brain is magnificent at substituting and

<hr>

formulating data that is missing. For me, that ability feels like it's been taken away. That then makes life difficult for others like family, friends and loved ones. They don't understand that missing ability in my brain. I wonder, do we really appreciate the magnificent power that we have within our brains? The brain builds/creates a version of reality based upon a mixture of sensory data, previous knowledge/conditioning/memory...and a vast array of unknowns.

When a localised area of the brain has been damaged (like through Stroke) it affects the entire brain....the brain operates like a collaborative global network not just a series of independent local networks. So when any of the network is missing (e.g. a localised fault), the entire global network is affected. Hello, welcome to my world.

What this does also mean, however, is that (given that we all create our own reality), I have the opportunity to create any future I choose!!!

Wow, that's amazing. This truly is an upgrade and reboot, but only if I want it to be!

I've started to capture this Reboot in a story...it's a story that charts the stroke, the recovery and the journey of redemption from the lessons from all this crazy experience called life.

I've started to pull this story together in an online format (ebook).

A preview of the first section will be available very soon.

So with that, today I choose to focus on the possibilities, heal

> *my faulty network and give myself grace and forgiveness when*
> *I miss my old self.*

The choice of thoughts determines one's reality. In every moment of every day, we have a choice, a choice of how or what we think. I finally figured this out in early January 2022. I had read this before and knew it academically but I didn't embody it, it wasn't a deep knowing in my core.

Then in January 2022 I finally realised that I could determine my future and craft it exactly the way I wanted. This was all part of the gift I had been given with the stroke. I hadn't been killed, I had survived. I had been affected, for sure. The world was a whole lot more dizzier now and even as I write this, my head still feels like it's full of cotton wool but I know those afflictions will eventually pass, they will simply go away and stop. I don't know when but I know they will if I think they will.

This was a huge and necessary shift in my consciousness. The way I thought about myself would determine...myself, wow, cool, this is powerful stuff right!?

It was also at this time that I fully realised that I would write this book. I knew it would be written. It might take a moment or it might take a moment. There was no deadline. I just had to get to work to make it happen and I wanted to produce a preview that people could read if they wanted. I knew how I could do that pretty easily and I made it available in an online (ebook) format.

Suddenly the world was full of possibilities, which of course it is. Life is all about possibilities and the experiences that we choose based on who we are, the thoughts and feelings we have, and the actions that we take.

In early January of 2022, that realisation was like a seismic shift in my thinking.

Transformation Key: The world is a playground of possibilities. Those possibilities can manifest in our experience through creative thought and feelings accompanied by aligned actions.

80

〰️

7 January 2021:
Depression Is Amazing,
Said No One, Ever!

Depression is amazing...

Said no one, ever!

It's only when I've lifted out of a period of absolute hell can I truly appreciate the contrast between light and dark.

I've often struggled with the dark winter months and general grey gloominess of the UK winter. I recall back in 2014 around Dec (and Christmas) I lost my job, my house and my (then) marriage and thought I was also going to lose access to my youngest kids too. It was a shitty time in my life and all within a single month.

Luckily I was to meet Claire a few months later who did her level best to make my birthday (Dec 21st) an amazing time from then on - trips to Corfe Castle, Rome, Edinburgh were all fantastic and made the former winter gloom disappear.

This year it returned with vengeance!

They do say that depression and mental illness are very common for Stroke survivors. OMG Yes, I can testify to that for sure! December was difficult for all manner of reasons which I won't divulge the details of here, but it culminated in my setback, loss of speech, increasing blood pressure, increasing imbalance and being blue-lighted into hospital on Christmas Eve, I also caught a heavy winter cold which seemed to knock me out and make all those new (and old) symptoms ten times worse.

So Christmas and New Year were awful and I felt extremely alone (mentally) and in my own dark place. If there was an easy way out, I would have taken that option. Luckily no such option crossed my path. I mean Jeez, I didn't survive this stroke just to then go and take my own life!!! What?! That doesn't make any sense right, but when you're in that dark dark place, all sorts of crazy shit comes into your twisted mind. In fact, it's the mind that creates those thoughts, the mind plays every kind of trick, trying to convince me that I have no future, no worth, no value...it's all BS but it seems so real at the time!

Luckily, somewhere, there remains a tiny spark of light. I managed to find it. Over the days following New Year, that spark has grown again.

Today, I've had two walks, one in the crisp morning air and this afternoon in the wet cold horrid weather with sleet and wet

snow falling and getting me soaked.
But I feel different. I feel lighter. I have a happier sense of self.
I feel optimistic. The light is burning brighter again (not fully
illuminated but brighter all the same)
So despite the current reality which is far from easy, today I
choose a sense of optimism and courage. Courage to lean into
the future with a greater sense of gratitude and a greater sense
of trust and faith.
I choose to walk with the light.
With love and light

I found that I could only post about depression once the feeling of depression had started to lift. When I was in the thick of it, I couldn't find the words to lift myself out of it. It had been a horrible time.

Having a Traumatic Brain Injury (TBI) for whatever reason (accident or ill-health like stroke) is so varied but one thing that I would say is common is the feeling of isolation. When someone has a broken leg, as bad as that is, there is a visible effect that everyone else can see and the brain is still working 'properly' (one would hope). With a brain injury I found that whilst I might have looked ok on the outside, I was not ok on the inside. I found that quite difficult to deal with. As I write this today, almost 10 months after the stroke, I still feel the effects with a continuous feeling of cotton wool in my head, constant imbalance when I stand and walk and my nose is blocked up and stuffy with a loss of smell. I suppose the difference today is that I don't let these things bother me so much and I just get on with life as best I can.

An aspect of feeling so depressed at that time was the sense of mental isolation, but the irony was that I sought physical isolation as a means of combating the depression. I find that interesting and I think everyone is unique in how they need to cope with themselves. As strange as this sounds, unique is a common characteristic of Stroke and TBI. Everyone is unique and every brain injury is unique and in that way, I suppose the thing that everyone else can do is simply monitor the situation without intruding. I know for me, had someone tried to force me out of the isolation and quiet that I yearned for, I would have been really upset and it might have made matters a lot worse. I had lost the ability to communicate clearly and my brain felt like fog so I would have hated it if someone tried to take control in that scenario. For another scenario, it might be entirely different and intervention might be the right answer. The secret is that there is "no one size fits all" solution. I can only thank the care and compassion of Claire once again that allowed me the space to be alone whilst I also knew she and her parents were on hand should I have felt the need to reach out.

As my depression lifted I did feel lighter. "Carrying the weight of the world" is a common saying, and feeling low can seem like a heavy burden to carry. These are all accurate metaphors and I have been there. I realised that I had been "carrying that weight" for years. In that early January 2022 period, I worked through some long-held emotional trauma.

In retrospect, perhaps it took me to become so utterly desperate and helpless to eventually find the deep-rooted emotional trauma of past hurt and pain. It would make sense. All I know is that since that time I have been different. I changed. There wasn't an immediate "ta-dah eureka" moment but more a gentle unfolding of a lighter-ness that started to take over my body and my mind. For want of another word, my heart had begun to fill with love for myself again and it felt such a relief. It was another gift from the stroke.

Transformation Key: When you are ready, your heart will begin to fill with love for yourself. This is a beautiful feeling and one to be cherished.

81

❦

8 January 2022: The Path Ahead

The Path Ahead is anything but clear.

Whilst the New Year is synonymous with goal setting, that seems like a long way off for me right now, but that is ok...I can only lean back with a state of trust and knowing that God will reveal the path when I'm ready. I am not even capable of "doing" anything at this moment anyway, so whilst it is completely alien to me, I have to just "be". Big goals will have to wait for the moment.

The daily walk around the woods is a great metaphor for life right now!!

The pathway is obscured and covered in mud; littered with obstacles; I slip; I slide, I wade through mud and rotten leaves, trying my best to stay upright and not fall on my face.

> *Yet despite the slipping and sliding, the way forward can suddenly be revealed.*
> *Not just that. Turn a corner, and then suddenly there are buds of new life pushing through!*
> *Nature has a way of showing me signs; showing what's possible when we leave it to take its own course.*
> *As I am incapable of taking specific action towards a future that resembles my past, I have to trust that (like the woods) the future will be revealed in a perfect way; a way that is better than anything I could design myself.*
> *A future that is perfect for me.*

Coming to terms with a completely uncertain future was a challenge that I had never fully had to do before. Having started up several businesses and taken risks, I had often faced challenging and uncertain times but this was entirely different. I had no choice in the matter. I had to accept my fate and that could have been scary as hell, but almost inexplicably, it wasn't. By confronting my fears and healing my past emotional trauma I now had an overwhelming feeling of calm take over my nervous system.

I had no idea what future lay ahead but I felt like I was going to be ok. Don't get me wrong, none of the craziness of life had disappeared, it was as uncertain as it could have been, but there was a new sense of peace even though nothing was certain, not even my ability to 'do' anything about situations and circumstances. I realised I just had to 'be' and not 'do'. It was the act of being that allowed inner peace and love to build within me. I think it's interesting that we are called human beings, not human doings. Perhaps we should spend more time being rather than just continuously do-ing, do-ing, do-ing.

Transformation Key: Be-Do-Have is one of the secrets to transformation. We must be the person we want to become and take the aligned action to have the rewards or benefits associated with that becoming.

82

〰️

9 January 2022: Do What Makes You Happy

Do what makes you happy.

I love doing and being in the moment...getting in the flow.

As I journey through my recovery, I can feel myself getting stronger and stronger every day.

The relapse over Christmas and New Year caused a setback in my ability to balance and my speech went really weird!!! My mental health took a knock too.

But, I really feel that is behind me now. My balance is still rubbish but I accept that and have a bit of a laugh at myself when I stagger a bit! I found my speech today is much better than before my relapse -yay!

I think this is helped by my ability to relax and do more of what I like.

> *This afternoon, I recycled some old candles and created a couple of new ones.*
> *I absolutely love working with candles and making new ones out of old burnt-out relics.*
> *I had the meditation playlist playing and my focus was on the wax and candle making.... I'm in my flow.*
> *So relaxing.*

Anita, Claire's mum. brought over some old candles that needed recycling. I had enjoyed candle recycling before the stroke so now was a perfect opportunity to do it again.

I enjoyed doing it. There was something deeply relaxing about the entire process from digging out the old candle wax to pouring the hot melted wax, it was all very therapeutic. I also played a meditation-type playlist which made the entire experience very peaceful and relaxing.

I was feeling confident that the depression and the relapse around Christmas had completely gone, I was building a strong recovery again and it felt good.

Transformation Key: Do what makes you happy. Being in your happy flow state will benefit your entire well-being.

83

12 January 2022:
New Days

New Days

What a stunning morning to be alive!

It might be cold; it might be muddy....

...but life is good. It feels like the perfect day to start over.

With an overwhelming feeling of knowing I am buzzing with ideas for my new business. I have the ideas for:

The name

The logo

The Products

The Collections

The Brand style

The Promotions

It's all pouring through me like gift after gift from Source. This state of knowing; this state of natural order; is all working in combination with my recovering body; my clearer mindset; my blood pressure medication and my mindfulness practices to produce a better version of me.

I know what I must create next. I'm excited about the unfolding of these next chapters. My blood pressure is dropping again. I know this is me.

I don't know what all this will look like exactly but that is ok, I feel the passion in my body. An entirely new direction that feels so very right.

I get so much inspiration from my natural surroundings near our home. I feel I am the luckiest person on earth to be exposed to such natural beauty. Every time I walk I feel reinvigorated and I return home bursting with ideas. The images on this post were taken on my walk this morning.

This natural beauty keeps me flowing with ideas; the natural order keeps me moving; it keeps me expanding to the next becoming, just like nature itself.

Here's to new becomings again and again and again - the continuous cycle of expansion and becoming.

Even though it was mid-winter and the woodland in which I walked daily was muddy and messy, I was now buzzing with life like I never felt before. Being out in nature was (and is) just the best feeling. The peace, the beauty, the energy, everything about nature is perfect.

Despite the mud and filth, I was able to see the beauty in

everything. As I relished in this natural beauty I also discovered that my ability to receive inspiration and downloads increased dramatically. Ideas and concepts were flying through my head. Very often I would have to stop my walk to capture the idea in a note on my phone. Capturing ideas with Notes on my phone has become a regular thing for me. I've now realised that if I don't capture the idea in the moment I could easily lose it from my memory. This is the same for remembering important events. I have to store all important events in the diary on my phone as well. So Notes and Calendar have been my primary go-to Apps on my phone post-stroke.

As I walked around the woods, I was getting idea after idea and inspiration was flowing through me in the bucket load, it was amazing to feel that way again. During that winter season in the woods, I could see the new life in the buds on the trees getting ready for the warmth of spring. It was an exciting time in the woods and it was an exciting time in my life, I was starting to fire on all cylinders despite my continued wobbliness and foggy head.

Transformation Key: Go to places that inspire you. When you're in those places (such as woodland or on the beach), notice the natural beauty all around you and use that beauty as a source of inspiration. Remember to make notes of the ideas and thoughts that come to you.

84

14 January 2022:
Brain Food

Brain Food

I'm at the stage in my recovery from a stroke where I'm getting stuck back into brain-building food again.

In the past, I'd never really been a fan of Blueberries but now they are just wow.

I made Claire and I Buckwheat and Banana pancakes for breakfast this morning.

As you can see, I love Blueberries now.

Blueberries are brilliant for the brain.

One of the worst things about the effects of stroke is the impact on the brain.

Brain damage is a horrible thing; almost indescribable tbh.

Imagine your brain as a heavy medicine ball inside your skull.

Now imagine that the medicine ball contains cotton wool. Now imagine moving around with the cotton wool heavy medicine ball inside your skull; it's heavy; it's slow; it's foggy; it lacks any form of clarity; it's a long way from being quick and nimble. Obviously, if the brain feels like that, now imagine what the rest of the body feels like!! Yep, it's not great. This is the best description of brain damage I can come up with at this moment.

But the most amazing thing about recovery is exactly that....recovery! Things are getting better.

Slowly but surely, taking one small step at a time, each day the medicine ball becomes less like cotton wool, it becomes a little lighter. The progress is painfully slow but there is progress and that is amazing.

Today I wrote in my journal these 3 entries under the heading, What Do I Choose To Believe?

1. God truly has my back
2. I can create plenty of passive wealth
3. I will continue to rebuild stronger and better than ever

Belief is everything. Belief will carry me over to the next point of expansion (recovery/rebuild).

...and those tiny little Blueberries? They all help.

Building new neurology is a constant process for every one of us whether we've had some form of TBI (Traumatic Brain Injury) or not. The brain is always adapting. In my quest to understand what foods would help my brain to build new neurology, I discovered that blueberries have incredible properties. I won't go into the details here but they contain flavonoids which are the real deal when it comes to brain cell production, memory and concentration.

I consume blueberries in every breakfast whether on pancakes, on my cereal, in my porridge, and always, in my daily smoothie.

When recovering from TBI such as the damage caused by a Stroke, the feeling in the head is very strange. It can be quite distressing. The most prominent symptom I experienced was a continuous feeling like cotton wool in my head which created numerous effects like foggy thinking, memory loss, unclear processing of certain data and various other effects that change from day to day, week to week and month to month.

One of the worst things about an injured brain is that no one can see it. The individual with the injury lives with it constantly. In that way, I have noticed that people treat me as if I'm perfectly well, which on the one hand is a good thing, whilst on the other hand, is quite difficult to deal with. That said, I subscribe to the school of thought that being treated like I'm perfectly okay might have helped in the speed of my recovery so far, so long may it last.

In my relationship with others, I was told in no uncertain terms by Claire to stop talking about the stroke. As much as it hurt my feelings at the time, she was right. She wasn't deliberately setting out to hurt my feelings but there were two main reasons: 1. the more I spoke about the stroke the more

I was feeding it power over me and recreating the ongoing symptoms, and 2. she had heard enough about it and didn't want the stroke to end up defining me in some way.

So as much as it felt a little harsh, in retrospect, Claire was right. If I kept on referencing back to the stroke then it would never be behind me, I could never just move on with my life. Some lessons are hard to hear sometimes but those are often the best lessons of all. My daughter, Charlotte, was the same. She also got tired of me linking things back to the stroke all the time, or drawing comparisons from something completely unrelated. She wasn't able to articulate it like Claire so I think Claire was speaking for Charlotte too. But that is all OK. They are correct, I have to move on with my life.

In respect of moving on with my life, a couple of working colleagues from the pre-stroke period reached out to me with offers of work that I could do on a part-time basis (e.g. 3 days a week). John contacted me in December 2021 and Tim in February 2022. I picked up contracts via both of these two amazing guys. I was so pleased that they had my back and thought of me. They both reached out on a similar basis. Both thought that getting back into some kind of work and contribution might help me and both were extremely sensitive to my recovery condition and did not want to put me under any strain or stress. The contract with Tim was for 35 days of work which I completed in May 2022, along with the creation of marketing blogs. The client with the 35-day contract was so pleased with the progress I had made that they allocated more time and budget to continue the work. I've been very pleased and I do think that being back in the world of work and feeling the satisfaction of contributing to a larger project has helped my recovery. As the saying goes, "God works in mysterious ways", and I do think that God had my back via these guys and these contracts. The pace of 3 days a week has suited me well. It has enabled me to combine self-care and recovery with brain stimulation and contribution to a larger cause whilst also allowing space for moments to write this book.

When considering foods to help with the brain, as well as the introduction of blueberries into my diet I have also introduced a daily dose of mixed seeds and omega-3 fish oil supplements. The mixed seeds are sunflower, pumpkin, hemp and flaxseed. I throw these into my daily smoothies at breakfast. When I researched these seeds I discovered that they contain omega-3. My theory is that if I can combine good sources of omega-3 and keep my brain stimulated then the chances of a healthy brain recovery are much better. With all that said, I still believe that the primary source of rebuilding strong neurology is linked to what I think and feel. In short, if I think I am well and I am in the process of building strong neurology, then I will, whereas if I don't think that, then I won't. This comes back to the basic rule of "you are what you think."

It is a hard concept to grasp. Well actually it's a simple concept to understand, but then actually consciously thinking in the right way can be hard to do. All manner of fears, doubts and sources of anxiety can creep in to disrupt any conscious effort to think in the right way. We have over 60000 thoughts per day so trying to stop the negative thoughts from slipping in is challenging. The majority of humans are also guilty of not thinking at all and running on autopilot. Yes, I am guilty as charged on this one and it's a very bad habit.

Transformation Key: "You are what you think." Instead of allowing your thoughts to run on autopilot try to consciously choose your thoughts to match the new reality that you are building for yourself.

85

16 January 2022: Getting
Better and Stronger

Getting better and stronger.

I feel heaps better and stronger than I did only 20 days ago!!

I spent the morning watching Will and his "Bassett" teammates secure two great victories over two solid opposing visiting sides in U13s rugby.

It was great to see Mark back at the club - we were chatting on the sidelines supporting our respective sons, just like in old times. Being able to do that again was a goal I set myself back in September last year when the Stroke hit....it felt amazing to be doing it again today, especially after the relapse I had at Christmas.

I must admit I was knackered when I got home so after a sofa snooze, Claire suggested we walk the dog as the sun was still up.

It was a beautiful sky as always.

We then all enjoyed a lovely roast dinner made by (mainly Claire) and I, followed by chess and jigsaw puzzle making (thank you Bryony, such a hard puzzle !!!)

At 10 pm the dog had been let out into the garden and returned to the house with exceptionally muddy feet!!

So Claire ended up washing his feet in the kitchen sink then Muggins here had to dry them off and lift him out!!!

None of that would have been possible months ago, even weeks ago!

My God, it's good to be alive

Being able to return to the rugby club to watch my son, Will, play again felt amazing to me. Of course, it was the same rugby club where the brain haemorrhage had occurred so the moment felt poignant in multiple ways. One of the first goals I had set myself when I was in the hospital and I had first discovered that I had survived an almost fatal brain haemorrhage just 7 months earlier was to get back to the rugby club and watch Will play again. Watching Will play brings me such joy and pride. He is so dedicated to the sport and trains almost constantly with the only exception being the summer months and break from the rugby season. So to be able to support him by physically being at matches once more, filled me with a renewed sense of pride and joy.

My eldest daughter, Bryony, of whom I am equally proud(I am proud of all our kids. They are all beautiful souls on their journeys), had kindly arranged for a jigsaw of Sydney harbour to be delivered for my birthday from her and her boyfriend Jack. Bry and Jack now live in the Bondi area of Sydney, Australia, and they are building an amazing life together. Bryony has conquered her fears to compete and win in multiple classes of bikini body-building competitions in Australia. I couldn't believe that I was seeing my firstborn baby girl when I saw the pictures of her competing in November 2021; she looked like a million dollars as she was doing her poses' and demonstrating the muscles that she had spent months and years developing and toning.

The jigsaw was a big hit with me and the family back home in England. It is 1000 pieces and hard with so much blue from the sea and the sky. It's good for the brain and a great reminder of Bry.

As it was still winter that meant rain, mud and limited daylight so letting Toby out into the garden before bedtime was rather a gamble to the state of his paws when he returned to be let back in the house. We always keep a collection of dog towels by the back door to wipe his feet before letting him back into the house. On some occasions even towels will not do the job of cleaning sufficiently so we have to wash them for him. Great! Wet muddy paws in the kitchen sink and just before bedtime, is not a great recipe for a relaxing end of the day and getting ready for bed and sleep. But living with Clare can be anything but boring. When she decides something needs to happen, it happens! It's not always a path I would choose but in the end, it is always worth the effort and upheaval; she is most often right. As I was still very much recovering, I didn't have much say in the matter anyway and just did what I was told (haha), so I happily obeyed the instructions and lifted Toby out of the kitchen sink to dry his wet feet before retiring to bed.

Transformation Key: Sometimes it's easier to move with the tide and join in rather than resist. Continual resistance can lead to a greater level of frustration, bitterness or anger which is not great.

86

⟨✦⟩

16 January 2022: The Foreground

The Foreground is treacherous; it might feel dangerous; unknown; challenging; risky; full of fears that seem to the mind to be very very real; scaring the heck out of me, but in the distance is the light; the warmth; the other side of the danger.

We seek the other side and get crazy scared of the things that lie in the way.

The here and now and immediate future appear to the mind as all disaster but holding a sense of knowing and trust in the midst of chaos is the key to letting the intuitive nudges come through; those gut feels; those moments of inspiration; those moments of clarity and the spark of imagination.

If I let fear grip me and run the show, I'll never feel; hear; sense; or imagine any of the new future. My mind will be clouded

> *with the fear.*
> *I breathe; I trust; I move forward at the pace my body will*
> *allow; I calm my mind and my nervous system.*
> *I breathe.*

Fear can have such power over us. I was at a point in my life and my recovery where I didn't have a clue what kind of destiny lay ahead; everything appeared to my logical mind as complete chaos. If I had let the fear rule then I could have easily attracted another serious ailment. Perhaps a heart attack, another stroke, Covid, cancer, who knows? The list is endless but the point is, I didn't let fear rule my thinking.

Every time I walked up to the woods in the early morning I would walk up the track which was frosty and frozen from the night and hadn't had the chance to thaw from the limited warmth from the winter sun. It is a magic time and the light from the morning sun fills me with joy and hope.

Feeling that sense of joy and hope permitted me to experience that light and love, and not perpetuate any feelings based on fear. I would swear in a court of law that experiencing that sense of love and beauty allowed me to simply relax and push aside any fears. Feeling fear in the form of doubts, worries and anxiety provides no value whatsoever. I had reached a point where worrying would not help the situation at all it might well have made the situation a whole lot worse.

People might say, but how can you not worry about paying

the bills or keeping the roof over your head? Don't get me wrong, there were many occasions where fear would take the driving seat but it was awful. It fucked me up to the point where I felt dangerously bad inside. My chest would tighten, my head would tense up, my breathing would become very shallow and numerous other signals all told me that my nervous system was running on fear and adrenalin. That is a very risky situation for someone like me recovering from a brain haemorrhage. Staying in that state for too long might have caused more burst blood vessels....er, no thanks!

There comes a point where surrender is the only option. I had reached that point. I had to trust in God and the Universe. I could feel a love that was reaching out to hold me and support me. I had no idea what lay ahead for me or our family. Claire was the most amazing person in that period. She was so grounded and didn't express her fears toward me at all.

We would journal together every morning to allow ourselves a specific and limited time slot to express our fears, hopes and beliefs. It was a magical time and we did the journaling exercise in such a way that we both felt heard and understood and that helped build a deeper trust in our relationship. We truly cared for each other's mental well-being.

Transformation Key: When it feels like God's plan is pushing you to breaking point, hang on in there and resist the temptation to let fear dominate your thinking. Try to see and feel the love and beauty in everything. It might be hard but it is there. When you feel the love you can also imagine a brighter future.

87

⟨✦⟩

17 January 2022:
Transition

Transition.

At 16:07 today (Jan 17, 2022) UK time, I was walking with Claire and our Toby dog and we were blessed to witness the simultaneous rising of the wolf full moon and the setting of the sun.

It was a spectacular moment that felt energising and lifted my spirit to a new height.

I've always been a mixture of earthy, and spiritual and feel a connection to all things...that's probably the most vague description ever but I don't care.

There are those that have a closed mind and those that have an open mind....I'm most definitely in the open-mind category...I don't dismiss anything....science can prove so much but there's still a huge amount of unknown so I lean towards possibilities rather than instant dismissal of the unproven.

I think that is why in moments like today/this afternoon I get very inspired and feel a great sense of oneness with the universe. Often I'll refer to God in my post. I don't mean God in the religious context, the God I refer to is a Universal Source Energy; a Divine Intelligence that is inexplicable but somehow stitches everything together.

It's in moments like today, and when I'm out in nature, that this God force is most apparent to me.

Folks might think I'm a bit barmy but quite frankly, I don't really care anymore. It's my truth and I'll stand by it.

So today I choose to praise Divine Intelligence for this magical celestial display.

What a moment to be alive

Being alive to witness a celestial display in our part of the physical universe is nothing short of miraculous. We often think of these moments and how they spiritually move us, but do we consider the miracles in everyday occurrences? That fact that we witness the Law of Attraction in action in our every moment and gravity being exerted all around us in the coordination of the planets in our solar system spinning in perfect timing and proximity to one another. Do we ever stop to consider this? Not often, I suppose.

Witnessing the rising of our moon whilst watching the setting of the sun in the winter sky is majestic. Imagine the kind of mind it must take to design the universe and all its magnificence with the timing and coordination of the gravitational forces on the moon and our planet circling the sun so that I could bear witness to that moment. I mean, wow, what a glorious thing!

The glory of the universe and the vast mind that moves in both huge and minute ways is so incredible that often as humans we ignore our perfection and place within the universe. We ignore that unlimited creative power that we have, that can forge any reality that we seek. I often refer to God when I consider this immense mind and the unlimited source of love that holds the universe together. I sometimes wonder if scientists will eventually discover that dark matter is in fact, love. Now there's a thought! I am convinced that through God's love (the invisible power that permeates the entire universe), I could choose and create a strong recovery and transcendent transformation of self that I chose to imagine for myself.

Transformation Key: Through the power of universal love it is possible to imagine whatever life we want for ourselves. We can imagine and feel that future in the heart, and then hold our patience with continuing trust and belief.

88

〰️

23 January 2022: From Hope To Knowing

From Hope to Knowing.

Earlier in my recovery journey I posted about finding and feeling hope for the future.

As I grow fitter and stronger with each day and learn to navigate the new version of me, I now move into a great sense of knowing:

Knowing that the future holds something amazing

Knowing that everything's going to be ok

Knowing that all of the lessons will be learned

Knowing that all of the hardship will have been worth it

As I continue to walk the woodland near home I can now see the early signs of the bluebells sprouting through the ground.

I know that the result of these shoots will be a spectacular show

---

of velvet flowers carpeting the entire woodland in April and May. It will be miraculous to behold.

Knowing is a great feeling.

With knowing comes a steadfastness that provides a guiding light like the stars that help navigate the lost ship at sea.

With knowing comes relief from the fears that can torment the mind but never the soul. The greater sense of knowing yields trust, belief and a wonderful appreciation of now, coupled with the momentum of the birthing of something truly great.

When the feeling of knowing is present it is such a profound sensation. Knowing is to embody a direction, a purpose of mind, a path that is lit up before you. It feels so sure.

The first sprouting of the bluebells in late January were signals that mimicked my knowing and reassurance of my recovery. The young bluebell shoots appearing from the warming earth below the insulating carpet of leaves from the previous Autumn signalled that spring was definitely on its way. Knowing that spring was around the corner helped fill my own heart with an equally powerful knowing that life was turning a corner for the better.

Transformation Key: When you find that sense of knowing you know that your transformation is starting to unfold for you. Bask in this glorious feeling.

89

⁂

24 January 2022: Candle Prototyping

Candle Prototyping

A whole new me...

...I spent this afternoon and this evening working on creating prototypes for my new candle company.

I have created a series of collections with the first collection prototypes being:

The Chakra Balancing Collection

The labels are in the design studio and yet to be printed, and the packaging boxes are also to be finalised, although I know what I want the packaging to look and feel like, I thought I'd share today's work to show what's brewing so far...

Exciting times but also very chilled and om.

So the new candle company was born. It was exciting. I love working with the candles and all the components that go into making a candle. Our kitchen provides a place for me to work and I find the entire process very relaxing and therapeutic. As I write this it is mid-summer 2022 and I paused the candle making for the summer months. I will pick it up again in the darker months of autumn and winter. My goal is to get the money together to buy a workshop for the garden where I can do the candle-making without relying on the kitchen.

I can picture in my mind's eye how the workshop will look and perhaps, more importantly, smell. My chilled-out playlist will be playing and I will have a small heater to keep off the cool air of those darker months of the year. It will be heavenly.

As I started with the candle making, it shifted from recycling old candles for fun to actively thinking up ideas for colour and fragrant combinations.

Given my love for all things spiritual, I fell in love with the idea of The Chakra Balancing collection as my first collection. As I tested different batches and quantities of ingredients (e.g. wax weight, size of tins, wicks, die colours, fragrances) I made meticulous notes, recording the results of each batch and test. I took a very scientific approach to the creations which suited my recovering brain perfectly. I realised that because my brain couldn't possibly keep track of all the different permutations and parameters, I had no choice but to keep detailed notes. I think that this has helped the process significantly because I know when I do return to candle making in the autumn and winter I can pick up my notes and continue from where I left off. This is a new side to my character. Before (pre-stroke) I might have rushed into it, got bored and moved on to something else (typical manifesting generator 1:3 profile in human design). This time, I've still moved on to other things which suit the summer months but I know I have my detailed notes when I return to it.

Transformation Key: Embrace the new you as 'you' emerge. Aspects of your character may have changed or been enhanced as you transform. This is normal and to be expected. This IS the point of transformation.

90

25 January 2022: Being Lit Up

Being lit up.

There's so much about this candle business that lights up my soul.

I find all aspects of the new business really fascinating and enjoyable.

Customer Experience

Creative Design

Manufacturing

Finishing

Cost Mgmt.

Packaging

Shipping

Supplies and Inventory

> *IT*
>
> *Mindset*
>
> *In my late teens/early twenties, I did an engineering apprentice-ship and that helped me learn from many departments in the manufacturing company. It's funny how running this new busi-ness reminds me of that time.*
>
> *Being involved in all of these aspects is fun!*
>
> *Today's news from the Manufacturing/Finishing process is that the colours are looking stronger today.*

As I went on my daily walks around the woods with Toby, I would find my mind wandering and thinking about the can-dles. I came up with ideas for different colours and fragrances and then arranged them in my mind into collections. In my mind's eye, I could imagine the collections in the packaging and how I would sell them at different craft fairs, country shows and online. I could "see" how it all would unfold, but all in good time, there was no rush.

First I had more testing to do. I wanted to try out different colours and dies and figure out how to get stronger colours and fragrances. It was around this time that I realised that my sense of smell was impacted by the damage to my brain. Later towards spring, I would use hay fever and pollen as an excuse for my lack of ability to smell but I don't think that is the case. But like everything, I will work on that ability and rebuild my sense of smell. It's not gone entirely, just certain fragrances and intensities.

As I wrote in the post that day, I enjoyed thinking about all aspects of the candle creations, ranging from the customer experience of buying, opening and lighting the candle through to packaging, design and the techniques I was learning to finish the candles in the manufacturing process. It was fun thinking about it all and as I carried out my tests I had made the detailed notes that would allow me to pick it all up again at a later date.

Transformation Key: When the ideas start to flow, find a way to capture them in a way that works for you. Some people keep a pen and paper close by, others might use their smartphone to capture notes or record voice notes. It doesn't matter what medium you prefer, but capture the ideas, because when they flow, they will flow fast!

91

26 January, 2022: ASD

ASD.

As I march on through this recovery from Stroke (almost 6 months ago!!) I am finding some interesting traits emerging/ re-emerging.

When I researched the traits of ASD for another person I started to recognise these traits in myself.

"OMG, that's me", I exclaimed, as I took the online test.

..and this is not just now, but also looking back on my past.

When looking back, I can recognise these traits and qualities in my past behaviour and I also recognise the stress from trying to mask those traits to fit in...it was so hard but for 53 years I had battled through....perhaps it was this underlying stress that caused my excessively high blood pressure...I was always pretty fit and healthy so the high BP made no sense to me or anyone else.

> *So now, as I progress with the recovery from Stroke and the inherent brain repair that is underway, I'm finding these ASD traits re-emerging.*
>
> *Research says that when an area of the brain is damaged, the entire network can be affected.*
>
> *This would explain a lot of what is currently in my reality but the great thing is, I'm just in a relaxed state of witnessing and acceptance.*
>
> *It's all part of The Gift.*

A significant part of the recovery journey was the self-discovery of who I am. This is ongoing and I've learnt to accept certain aspects of my character as "just who I am" rather than resisting or fighting those things.

As a backstory to this particular aspect, I was doing some research into ASD (Autism Spectrum Disorder) concerning another younger family member. It was another challenge for our family, and we had to learn very quickly how to manage one of our children, which impacted each of us in the family. It was a period when I had to accept that I was on my recovery journey alone. I realised that my recovery was de-prioritised. That was difficult for me to accept at the time but I had no choice, every member of the family had to adjust and I was no exception. On reflection, it was a positive sign that my recovery was going well and that I was able to be 'de-prioritised'. Given that this particular situation concerned the well-being of one of our children, it was only right to step back and deal with my recovery alone for a while.

As I researched online about different forms of neurodiversity like ASD, ADHD, Dyslexia, Dyspraxia etc., I realised that when I read about the traits and characteristics of ASD, ADHD and Dyslexia, I thought, "This is me!"

I took an online test for ASD and Dyslexia and sure enough, I scored as moderate ASD and mild Dyslexia. Since reading more about the characteristics of ADHD, I am tempted to take that test as well. I'm not that concerned about getting an official diagnosis but I did find that discovering and labelling these aspects of my character both relieving and revealing. "So I'm not strange after all!", was my general response to myself in my thoughts. Being moderate ASD and mild Dyslexia (and I wouldn't be surprised if was moderate ADHD as well), was kind of comforting in a strange way, in so far that I wasn't alone; this was a big relief for me and it explained an awful lot of my behaviour patterns of the past.

I'm pretty sure that my recovering stroke brain has a lot to do with my current traits so I don't want to get a misdiagnosis. I would say that a recovering brain injury might display traits similar to ASD and ADHD. For instance, my immediate short-term memory is not at all good and therefore my ability to multitask has been severely affected; in short, I forget what I'm doing if I am not vigilant. This could be linked to ADHD, so I look at it as another thing to work on and build in my recovery. I have always found the ability to concentrate on a single task incredibly difficult and I work in short bursts of energy.

Even the writing of this book has taken months because of distractions. I have always 'flitted' from topic to topic and interest to interest. I used to think there was something wrong with me. But now, I accept it as one of my characteristics and love it. I'm interested in so many different things; I always have been. I used to get annoyed by my lack of focus to concentrate on a given task, but having accepted it as just a part of my character, I have strangely mastered the ability to focus much more. This is a strange (unexpected) outcome which I find fascinating. So the more I resisted my former behaviour and distractions the worse it seemed to be, whereas now I've accepted and embraced it, the more focused I've become.

Transformation Key: Love who you are and embrace your characteristics. The greater resistance you build up about yourself, the more that unwanted behaviour will reveal itself. Relax and love all of who you are.

92

***

26 January, 2022:
Milestones

Milestones.

I used to miss the little things...they used to pass me by without a second thought....not present perhaps?

This evening I went to the rugby clubhouse of RWBRFC with Roger as my son did his Wednesday training with his U13 teammates.

So the last time I had a pint of Thatchers Haze from the clubhouse was the moment (6 months ago) that the brain haemorrhage struck!

It's not an understatement to say that was quite a life-changing moment!

So sitting in the clubhouse drinking this pint was a massive milestone.

I'm not a big drinker so the point is not the cider, the point here is being present, the milestone and the fact that I am alive and recovered enough to actually do this at all.
So rather than drinking the pint without any real thought, this moment meant everything to me!
Cheers

I am writing this whilst sitting in the rugby clubhouse again. However, I am now tee-total. Mine is a pint of lime and soda and not the cider like I used to have. As well as being nice and refreshing it's a lot cheaper too!

After this post in January, I would have a pint every week but I realised that I was doing it out of habit rather than enjoying the pint, so I decided I don't need or want alcohol in my life anymore, it's as simple as that.

Getting back to the rugby club where the brain haemorrhage had occurred was a big deal and to taste a cider again was an even bigger deal. The senses (including smell and taste) will invoke emotions and memories, some of which can be very deep. Sitting inside the clubhouse drinking my cider could easily have brought up some disturbing feelings but it passed by without any trauma and resurfacing of emotions of sadness, anger or frustration. It was all very 'normal' as if nothing had happened 6 months earlier. I suppose that is also a reflection of the friends at the rugby club. There was compassion and care of course, but there was also a very grounding sense of normality and business as usual that made the situation very 'safe'.

Transformation Key: Do the things that you might think scare you. When you face your fears and do the things that you think might trigger you, you might be surprised that the situation will be fine and any fear will immediately dissipate.

93

27 January, 2022: Taking Strides

Taking Strides.

Almost 6 months ago when the blood seeped into the cerebellum of my brain I was completely and 100% reliant on Claire for physically supporting me as we walked back across the field of the rugby club towards our car where we had parked.

I was a physical wreck and life was changing in that moment in a huge way!! I couldn't walk. I was staggering as my vision was literally turning everything upside down and round and round....it was a living hell that I would not wish upon any-one, ever.

As I think back to that moment and the days immediately after the stroke, and then look at the strides I take today as I walk across the fields near our home, I am reminded of the incredible ability of the brain to undertake its own repair.

The dizziness and unsteadiness are still there in almost every moment but I'm coping with it and I know one day it will be gone.

This morning I walked alongside Claire roughly 6 feet apart. I walked with determination and drive. If only the hospital physio team could see me now!?

Claire said, " So if you're this good after 6 months, what are you going to be like after another 6 months?"

This journey is anything but fast and the day-by-day progress seems unbearable on some days.

But, when I zoom out and look at the big picture, the progress has been remarkable.

My daily exercise routines include:

Yoga x 2 (morning and night)

Press Ups x 50 (morning and night)

Walking x 2 (through woods and fields)

There is no way on earth that those exercises could be accomplished until now.

No matter how bad you think it is (pick another form of recovery)....in the end, it will get better. The body is an amazing healing machine....it just needs time, care and patience.

Have a great day

When you undertake a huge transformation (in my case

a transformation based on recovery and awakening) it is remarkable how the the human brain can rebuild.

In the moment of day after day of tedious repetition, it feels like there is no change, no transformation at all. It was only when I found the perspective to zoom out and look at the whole journey it became apparent how far I had come.

When I wrote this post on 27 Jan, 2022 I was 6 months post-stroke. As I sit and write this it is now over 10.5 months post-stroke, I recall that earlier today I was climbing a stack of pallets to select, shift and transport pallets from a building materials yard to our back garden to construct a pallet-based garden sofa. All of this seemed so distant when the stroke occurred but we (you/me/anyone) can do anything we set our minds to if we want. Was I thinking about climbing a stack of pallets in the early days of stroke recovery? Well, funnily enough, no. But the point is when you persevere and stick to the repetitive things that seem like they are doing no good whatsoever, you will find that remarkable transformation has been and continues to be taking place.

If someone had suggested during October 2021 that I would be climbing a stack of pallets 10 months later I would have laughed at them.

As I've said numerous times throughout this book, everything starts in the mind. Everything starts with imagination. Our ability to create is unquestionable and we can create anything we want. The trouble is we let doubt and fear stop that creativity, so the vision is just a distant memory and dream which causes more frustration and self-doubt, proving to ourselves that great things only happen to other people.

Bullshit! Sorry, but it's true. Utter BS. Anyone can do anything if they want. Humankind would dream of flying or walking on the moon, running a mile in 4 minutes, or ... keep going...every achievement, every invention, every single human-made thing has once started in the mind of a person. As Human Beings, we are blessed creatures with the power of the universe coursing through our veins. We can do anything. This is not wishful thinking or pseudoscience. If you wish to research the science read anything by Dr. Joe Dispenza. I am also proof that the ability to heal and recover is possible but what I can also add is that, in my case, the process has involved a deep spiritual awakening and transcendence. If that is not your thing then that's ok maybe it's time to put down this book until a moment later in your life. I bid you farewell and good luck with your journey. For those of you still here, let's continue.

So every accomplishment from brain recovery and healing to walking on the moon starts with a vision in the imagination. This is the seed of all expansion in the universe. Creating anything is expanding the universe (both metaphysical and physical). Every idea and every thought in imagination expands the spiritual universe. Whether that thought is good or bad the expansion takes place, so we have to be very mindful of what thoughts we place our attention on and those thoughts we don't place our attention on. It's our subconscious thoughts that often run the show and continuously create our reality. Those thought patterns that are habitual and almost programmed into us. Those carry just as much power as good thoughts, so try hard to become more aware of your thinking.

Being hit by a stroke completely out of the blue is a very testing time (physically, mentally, emotionally and spiritually). I was tested "to the max" and somehow through the unconditional love from Claire and the unconditional love I found for myself, I have found a pathway through the chaos.

I am not "out of the woods' yet but I know I am getting stronger and stronger all the time. I have reached a point in my recovery where I can send out unconditional love to others. I am a member of several stroke-related social media groups and I will regularly contribute with my posts of inspiration and comment on other people's posts who are having a difficult time. My sole/soul purpose in this contribution is to give back. I mean give love back, or give love out. There are many suffering and if I can help in my way then that has got to be a good thing, right?

I remember my late father saying to me and Claire in a visit to our home before the various lockdowns of 2020/2021, he said, "I've figured out that our purpose on this planet is to help others." No more. That was it. I think he was spot-on. It makes me very proud to continue that legacy.

Transformation Key: All transformation starts in the imagination with thoughts and ideas. All thoughts expand the spiritual universe so try hard to become aware of your thoughts. Think thoughts of love to expand the universe in a loving way.

94

⚜

29 January, 2022: Helping Others

Helping Others.

This evening I was able to offer advice to another survivor of stroke going through a tough time in her recovery.

I saw her post on a Stroke website and wrote this message:

"Hello <name> - it is been almost 6 months since I survived a brain haemorrhage in the cerebellum area of my brain. I know exactly how you feel with disorientation and balance problems.

I have found that in order to help my brain build new neurology and pathways I do physio that causes a mild version of the symptoms and then stop and let the symptoms settle....then repeat, do the exercise, cause the symptoms and stop to settle again. Building new pathways is analogous to the building of new roads to complete a journey because the old roads are broken. The new roads need carving out of fresh earth. The new pathways need to be established for the "normal" function to be re-established. Unfortunately, other parts of the brain don't like this new building of these pathways and then send other signals to the body to cause disorientation, vertigo, dizziness....in fact, anything to cause us to stop. When those symptoms get bad stop and settle. This will teach the brain new patterns and pathways. This approach works. No medication is necessary just basic physiotherapy, persistence, patience....and a lot of self-love....it's a long journey with no quick fix (I'm sorry) but you will get better I promise.

On the bad days when I've felt really down and sorry for myself (which is ok btw), I just focus on the fact that I/we/you are on the journey to recovery... it may be long but it's still recovery.

Sending you love and support

Simon"

I sincerely hope that <name> gets some hope and comfort from my experience and advice.

I've always managed to get on with people. It's because I'm interested in people and want to help wherever I can apply my skills and knowledge. That said, I've generally been pretty rubbish at 'selling myself' but my demeanour has always been friendly, positive and forthcoming.

A various points in my recovery journey I have browsed and contributed to various websites and forums focused on survivors of stroke.

In recent months (since June 2022) I've been a member of a Facebook group linked to the UK charity, Different Strokes. The group is of the same name and it contains 6700+ members (at the time of writing), all of whom are either survivors of stroke or related to survivors of stroke. It's a wonderful group with all members offering support and compassion to one another by reading and commenting on each other's posts.

As I have been so fortunate with my recovery, I feel in a strong place to be able to offer my support, compassion and advice when I feel it's appropriate or when I'm inspired to do so. I also post messages about my more recent recovery milestones and landmarks as a source of inspiration and hope for others.

I am always very positive and send out love as I know first-hand how utterly scary having a stroke can leave a survivor and their family.

I have noticed another related attribute of myself that I'm proud of and it has come to the surface during my recovery, and that is my ability to connect and speak to those with mobility, neurodiversity or debilitating issues. I find I can speak my truth and speak to everyone normally. I know it may sound awful to say, but I couldn't do that as my former self, and I would shy away not knowing what to say, and feeling slightly awkward. These days, having had brain damage myself, I feel no barriers whatsoever and can approach people who just want to be treated normally and as a normal human being, despite any difficulty, impairment or difference.

To elaborate on this new aspect of my character that I love, I have been welcomed into Sailability within a wonderful local sailing club.

Every Wednesday, I now go to Sailability and sail a Hansa 303 dinghy sailing boat (dinghy class), single-handedly. I have also gained my RYA Level 1 - Start Sailing certification which can help me towards a new goal of racing a Hansa 303. Only today, I signed up for racing training at the club and most of these people (if not all) are either part of or enjoy Sailability. The point here is that having the stroke has opened up new areas of life and this is wonderful. None of this would have happened if it wasn't for Claire, her family and the kind people at Sailability at the Whitefriars Sailing Club in South Cerney.

It was Claire who wanted to pursue her lifelong passion for water sports and sailing, and so one weekend she said to me, "I've found a sailing club near us. Let's take a look." She contacted the club and low and behold we were then visiting the club on a lovely sunny Saturday afternoon in the height of the Summer. We spoke to a kind man called Rupert who seemed to know what he was talking about, although I must admit I was as confused as hell. Sailing had never been my thing and being candid, I wasn't that interested in the thought of sailing. So there we were, chatting away and before I knew it, we'd told Rupert all about me having a stroke and he said, "Well, don't let that stop you! Come on down to Sailability." He went on to explain how Sailability worked and then that was it, Claire was signing me up for Sailability and her brother Lee generously paid for a year's family membership at the club. Wow! When the universe moves it moves fast and all the pieces of the puzzle drop into place.

Transformation Key: Sometimes the universe can move us and deliver to us things that we could never plan ourselves and all we have to do is be willing to graciously receive with thankful hearts.

95

30 January, 2022: Grit

Grit.

Grit is a very masculine energy. I don't mean macho, I mean it's an energy that is the embodiment of drive, determination and progression.

I'm a human who fully embraces my feminine energy. That doesn't mean I'm feminine, I don't think, or maybe it does (I don't care what anyone thinks tbh).

Balance is the key in my opinion. I embrace both masculine and feminine energies.

So back to Grit.

As I think back to this journey of recovery over the past 6 months I realise that it has taken (and still is taking) a true balance of masculine and feminine energies to heal and grow stronger. A major factor has been the ability to tap into the masculine energy of grit.

That said, if it was all grit, push and determination then the recovery would not have been anywhere near as strong. I'll say it again, it's all about balance....the yin and the yang.

If I had taken a total lean-back approach and said I'll let time (alone) do the healing then that might work (I think) but not as effectively. Recovery from brain damage is a very weird thing. On the outside I think people look at me and think he's ok he can do x or y. Actually inside the brain is having a hard time figuring out what is x or y, x and y, x nor y.....it gets confused....at everything.

But grit and determination balanced with self-care and love help to build a new brain that each and every day is just that little less confused.

When I hear of stories about others having stroke I am totally amazed and chuffed to bits (very happy) with my recovery. I find myself in complete empathy with anyone having brain injury or any form of brain degenerative disease. To be lost in your own head is horrible but for me and my personal journey, I know that my condition will ultimately get better and a completely new version of me will emerge....how f...ing cool is that??? Wow!!!

I would never have thought that this journey would be so fascinating.

Forever the nerd.

So there we have it, perhaps this post summed up the secret to my recovery...balance. How ironic that balance is the secret and yet balance was/is the primary function within my brain that got slammed by the stroke! Isn't that interesting (well it is to me)? This post from the end of January 2022, just 5.5 months after the stroke, showed that I had figured out, even after that short time (short in stroke recovery terms) that I was getting better. I knew and was confident about the path I was on.

How did I know? I just knew. I didn't need validation from any doctor or medical professional. I trusted in a much higher power and that power came through for me like a good 'un.

As the post suggests, it takes balance to thrive in this universe. The balance of energies (masculine and feminine) and I don't mean men and women, I mean energies.

I've heard a great metaphor using water to describe the difference between masculine and feminine energies which I will borrow but I am in no way taking credit from this metaphor (although I wish I could as it's that good!) So, when you think about water in terms of a flood this is like feminine energy. Now imagine river banks, that is masculine energy. It is the combination of the water and the river banks working together that creates the power from the channelled and directed water (i.e. the river).

One energy without the other, doesn't necessarily serve a purpose, whereas the combination of both can be used to great effect and purpose and the combined energy can be converted into other energy.

Transformation Key: It is the combination of masculine and feminine energy working together in harmony that yields incredible results.

96

31 January 2022: Emotional Intelligence

Emotional Intelligence.

Yesterday's post about the energy of having grit and determina-tion is completely at odds with today's overriding feeling I have of sadness.

I realise how I perceive reality and particular circumstances are based entirely on the emotions I hold in my body.

As sadness comes up in today's reality I decide to allow myself to move into a place of self-care and forgiveness. For me, this transition into self-care and forgiveness has a feminine energetic signature. It feels good to me at this moment.

The other interesting aspect of this is that in addition to the sadness, I also sense a small light of love.

The dualities are profound and this is what I was referring to in yesterday's post with the Yin and Yang energies. E.g.. From Grit to Sadness; from Sadness to Love.

We all feel these mixed emotions. This is normal and totally ok. Although many people often suppress the emotions that don't feel good....I used to too. Now I just feel it. I've learnt from my partner, lover and the wisest oracle I know, Claire that holding onto these emotions and giving them meaning (i.e. if this <emotion> then that <meaning>) serves no purpose and benefit whatsoever. Releasing the emotion safely (eg. it's ok to cry when feeling sad) is an amazing toolset to understand the lessons and help reach the other side of the emotion. I choose to feel the feelings, without any meaning and then release them with forgiveness and love for myself. Yes this means I might ball my eyes out, and not really know why, and that's ok....it's time for the sadness to come out.

Ultimately, I choose to believe that all there is is love. I'd say that even hate is a form/version of love. So the emotions and dualities I experience in any given moment are merely expressions of love. I believe that when the sadness clears it then reveals more of the love (like fog clearing to reveal a stunning vista)

I've come across many articles and books written about Emotional Intelligence but very few (if any) of those that I've read dig into the level and mastery of Emotional Intelligence that I had to experience during my recovery.

I attribute this mastery to the wisest teacher of this subject that I have ever known, my partner, Claire. Without Claire at my side, I'm not sure I would have learnt this level of profound understanding, but as I look back on this post of January 2022, I am re-learning the nuances of Emotional Intelligence all over again.

This statement from the end of the post is profound so I'll state it again:

"Ultimately, I choose to believe that all there is is love. I'd say that even hate is a form/version of love. So the emotions and dualities I experience in any given moment are merely expressions of love. I believe that when the sadness clears it then reveals more of the love (like fog clearing to reveal a stunning vista)"

Wow, this is a huge statement and so right.

If one truly believes (like I do) that there is only love in the universe, then everything in the universe is an expression of love. It has to be that way. Many people will argue that all the harm and wars that happen in the world are anything but an expression of love and with the human construct and definition of love that would be a correct assumption. But at the level of love at the universal level is that true?

From my own experience, when I came to release any 'negative' feeling or meaning associated with an emotion, I felt liberated. I think about love as a continuum with the human understanding of love at one end and the human understanding of hate at the other. Now imagine along every point on that continuum is some expression of love, but the whole continuum represents love. Now it is possible to see that hate is an expression of love. Of course, no one wants to experience that polar opposite of human love, but as a means to process 'negative' emotions, thinking about every emotion being an expression of love does help. Notice that I also place the word 'negative' within quotation marks. That is deliberate because as humans we assign a 'negative' meaning to 'bad' emotions. All this 'negative' and 'bad' is made up by our human selves as a means to try to understand the emotion. Why do we do that? It serves no useful purpose. How about the emotion just is? It just is and let's leave it at that! Perhaps assigning some kind of meaning or label serves no one at all. Assigning a meaning could even perpetuate the emotion and keep it trapped within us when the best, and most fruitful, thing to do is to just feel the emotion as it is (finally) released from the body. The process of feeling the emotion (let's say sadness) is to feel the emotion and then let the accompanying tears flow. When I discovered the ability to do this myself, I found it the most liberating thing I could ever do for myself

Transformation Key: Mastery of Advanced Emotional Intelligence is one of the most powerful tools for self-actualisation and transformation.

97

1 February 2022: An
Appeal For Help Please

An appeal for help, please.

Hello,

Could anyone connect me with book publishers, please?

I have completed the first 3000+ words of my forthcoming book to capture my personal story of Stroke Survival, Recovery and Rebirth of my life.

My hope is that other Stroke Survivors can benefit from my story. Did you know that every year 795000 people in the US have a stroke? In the US, someone has a stroke every 40 seconds! It's a horrible condition and the resulting recovery from the brain damage is very difficult. My wish is to ease the suffering as best I can.

I feel the book is now at a point where someone in the publishing

> *world would benefit from seeing where this can go. I would esti-*
> *mate that at 3000+ words I am approximately 1/6 distance.*
> *Thank you in advance for any help/connections/introductions*
> *My sincerest thanks*

So the book writing was well underway! It's funny as I write this now. I imagined at the time when I wrote that post on Facebook asking for help that at 3000 words I was 1/6 or about 17% through the book. As I write this I can see that the word count is 68027, which is far more than the almost 18000 words that I thought it would take, and we're not finished yet!

I truly hope you're enjoying this journey through these months of my life and that you're able to learn from my experience.

You may have noticed that each narrative of each diary entry is followed by a Transformation Key, and you may be asking yourself why.

Over the last 5 years, I've read a lot of self-development books and I've been on my journey of self-actualisation and becoming. It's been more than that, I'd describe it as a journey of remembering. Remembering who I truly am at the deep, spiritual and soul level.

So why the Transformation Keys? Well, I see the events that happen to me as all happening for me, never to me. The events, the lessons, and the wisdom that I have grown to understand have all been so that I can truly remember my spiritual self and become the true me that I was originally born to be. This is a gift and so, in turn, my gift is to pass that on to others who can also learn and grow to understand perhaps without having to go on the journey that I went on. Even if someone also had a stroke and went on a similar journey, they would never actually go on the same journey because they would go on their own unique journey. We are all here following our own journey and soul path to learn the lessons we are here to learn before leaving. The Transformation Keys is a set of lessons that might help and guide others.

Transformation Key: Every lesson that we learn on our soul path could help someone else; always consider how your lessons could help others.

98

1 February, 2022: Tears Of Joy

Tears of Joy...are truly amazing.

Probably for the first time in my life, I've finally experienced tears of pure joy.

People often use the expression and sure, I've experienced tears with laughter before but this was something entirely different.

As I walked out with Toby dog this afternoon and we walked into our favourite field, I glanced across to my right to the western sky as the late winter sun was setting.

Wow, the moment brought me to tears

I had an overwhelming feeling of gratitude to be nothing more than alive at that moment.

I've been working on my book earlier today and recalling the moments when I had the stroke and my initial recovery journey.

> *I think this hit home again for me today while I was out walking, but this sense of joyful gratitude was like nothing I'd ever experienced before.*
>
> *The magic of being alive to witness that specific moment was profoundly special.*
>
> *Next time you are served up a sight that takes your breath away stop for a moment to give thanks to a vast intelligence that we get to be a part of and witness.*

If I haven't already mentioned it, I am truly blessed to live in a part of the world that is truly beautiful. When I first moved into the area and started living with Claire and her family in 2015 I had a great sense of gratitude for where we lived but as I had spent so much time in recovery during the latter part of 2021 and into 2022, the beauty and splendour of the world became so clear to me.

Given that I had also been through some profound emotional healing during the end of January 2022, I could then perceive the world in a way that felt more... well more everything really. More colourful, more beautiful, more majestic, more stunning, more intelligent, more peaceful, more possibilities, everything just felt more alive. As I started to perceive this more-ness of the world and my gratitude for being alive grew and grew the tears would flow, and the only way to describe those tears were tears of deep and utter profound joy.

Transformation Key: Never take anything for granted. Develop a deep sense of gratitude for everything in your world. Not a superficial surface-level appreciation but a gratitude that is an outpouring of love from your heart.

99

2 February, 2022: Helping Others

Helping Others.

As this phase of my recovery journey unfolds, it's becoming more and more clear that my overriding purpose moving forward is to help others who have sustained brain injury.

With so many people in the world having Strokes (young and old and everything in between) and with other types of brain injury, the need for helping others is vast.

As I think about my own recovery and my gratitude for my physical abilities, I am constantly reminded of my own brain injury which (of course) no one can see.

Having experienced (and still experiencing) this first-hand, I hear about others with brain injury and think to myself, "I understand them!"

The feeling of confusion and being lost in your own head is in-describable. I've used words like foggy or numbness as a means to describe it but nothing quite hits the mark. As I walked in the sunlight this afternoon, I realised that helping others with Stroke and brain injury is my path. This will include my books and my Candle creations, but it will also be something else...

...I'm not sure what yet, but it will reveal itself in good time, I'm sure.

For now, if anyone knows or hears of anyone else having a Stroke please let me know and pass on my contact details.

Stroke is unique in every case but the commonality of brain injury is universal. I'm here for a chat/messaging/support for anyone who needs it.

I'm sure I am repeating myself, but as I've found strength in my own recovery, I try to help others by shining a light on what is possible. I don't wish to make out that I'm some kind of miracle or miracle worker, but if I can help others through my positivity then that seems like a good thing to me.

Sustaining a brain injury is horrible. No one can dress it up any other way. One of the most difficult things that I find is my own state of anxiety about what I think people are thinking. Oh boy, what a waste of energy that is and it's so damn easy to disappear down the rabbit hole with that sort of thing. For example, I can sometimes get lost thinking that people think I'm ok and treat me as if I have a fully recovered brain, whereas inside I'm still working with my imbalance and weirdness, even after 11 months since the stroke.

But with all that said, I know that I am very fortunate and have made a remarkable recovery so far in such a (relatively) short period of time.

One of the things that I must stress is that every occurrence of stroke is unique. Sometimes (often) it can be fatal and other times the symptoms are hardly noticeable. A brain haemorrhage like I had is often very bad news indeed, but here I am 11 months after experiencing such a massive event, still writing this book. My point is that each survivor is unique and no one must judge themselves by comparing themselves to me or anyone else. Like I say, "I am not out of the woods yet" but I am able to function independently and in the past 4 months I have been able to do part-time work and earn a living to help financially support our family. I can do so much and I'm even considering returning to the gym to get back in shape. Of course, any return to the gym will be accompanied by very careful monitoring of my blood pressure.

Transformation Key: If your life has been literally "turned upside-down", it can become the catalyst and opportunity to become more than you ever previously imagined.

100

4 February 2022: Zip a dee doo dah, Zip a dee ay

Zip a dee doo dah, Zip a dee ay...My, oh my, what a wonderful day!

Plenty of sunshine, headin' my way

Zip a dee doo dah, Zip a dee ay!

This morning during my morning yoga I started singing this famous Disney movie song!!

No idea why, but boy I felt great.

My 15-year-old daughter looked at me with that "What the hell do you look like?" Look, like 15-year-old daughters do.

I didn't care. As I stretched and went into my poses and reached for the sky, I just carried on singing!

...and what a great day it's turned out to be for me.

For the first time in 6 months, I felt truly able to emotionally hold my Claire. She's held it all together as the family has gone through absolute shit in the last 3 months and of course my (so far) 6 month recovery from stroke.

She needed holding today and I said "Baby don't do anything today, I've got you." It felt good to say that again and mean it.

Also, my favourite customer gave me a 10/10 for my first piece of marketing content. He (the MD) and his chairman really valued my work and he then published it straight away on social media.

We then talked this afternoon and there's plenty more content to be done and a full customer assessment could be on the cards too.

Another favourite customer contacted me to ask for an estimate for some other work too.

Now I'm in the kitchen preparing a healthy dinner for Claire and I before we settle to watch something cool on the TV tonight. I expect she'll get a foot rub too.

Onwards and upwards.

It felt so unbelievably good to feel like I was really starting to return to my former self again. For 5 months I had been lost. Lost in my recovery, lost in rebuilding my brain from the ground up, lost in the depth of the depression, lost in the ramifications of a stroke that had been thrown my way in what felt like an indiscriminate and chaotic manner. To start to feel like my 'old' self again was the manifestation of the turning point that started in January. Of course, this was just another phase and chapter in the recovery process.

One day and no one can predict when this will happen, but one day, things will start to get better. When someone feels the state of utter despair that precedes the feeling of euphoria it seems that this feeling would be impossible; one can easily think that everything is lost but one day the glimmer of hope starts to burn a bit brighter.

This is a bit like a sports team playing against a tough opposition. Momentum can change in the game, and when that happens it can be the deciding factor between winning or losing. Momentum carries a lot of power in any sport and so it is with transformation and healing too.

Success builds success. Once I felt the tide turning in my favour, I was able to build on that change of fortune; that shift in momentum and build upon different areas of my life.

I secured a contract with and via some great working colleagues from my pre-stroke days. Both Tim and John individually had my back and I was so grateful. Both (almost simultaneously) made contact with me to see if I was feeling ok to do some work. Both guys were working with other customers but they both thought that I would be suitable to undertake specific aspects of each respective contract. I felt confident and able to take on both contracts and looked forward to getting started.

I also took on a part-time role creating marketing content for Tim and his company. He runs a successful consulting company which keeps him fairly busy, in fact too busy to focus on marketing content like blogs to keep his company in the forefront of leadership thinking. Given that my background was in the same industry and I was a global leader in a software in that same industry, Tim thought that it might help us both if my skills and knowledge could be put to use. He was incredibly understanding and said that I could work at my own pace with zero deadlines or pressure. Of course, I accepted the challenge and couldn't wait to get started.

It is now mid-August, 2022 as I write this and my contracts with Tim and the customers linked to both Tim and John are continuing. When I look at the benefits from these contracts, the list is substantial. But if I had to put my finger on the top three benefits of this work it would have to be:

1. Money. Yes, being able to pay the bills and plan for future expenditures (birthdays, parties, family events etc.) has been a massive relief to my nervous system and levels of stress. In the deepest part of my depression from November and December, I think one of the primary contributing factors was my inability to do anything about being able to address our family's financial situation. It scared the crap out of me. Claire was brilliant during that time. She had successfully kept our heads above water (financially) in the early months of my recovery through her own coaching business but she had become distracted (not surprisingly) with the sudden switch to adapt to homeschooling and managing ASD triggers in our youngest boy, coping with an emotional wreak of a recovery stroke patient (aka me), and providing emotional support to our daughter/

step-daughter...and I could add more to that list. Life was anything but easy, and she was keeping all of that together whilst all I could do was focus on my recovery. So something had to give at that time, and it was financial security that scared the bejeebers out of me. Our home expenses were continuous and rising, but the income had disappeared completely. Whilst I freaked out and worried about keeping our home, Claire kept a very cool head and instilled an amazing sense of calm about the situation. She helped us through that storm with such grace and poise. We would journal together every morning to allow ourselves to express our deepest fears. It was a brilliant routine that helped. Claire taught me so many incredible tools and techniques for managing mental health and stress, I love her so much. Words cannot describe the depth of my love for Claire. She was (and is) the rock of the family. For me, being able to finally address financial security was a huge win for us all. It felt like we were thriving again and I was contributing to the success of the family once again. We were, and are, a team in every sense of the word.

2. Contribution. I have great pride in doing a good job and being able to go above and beyond if its appropriate to do so. With these contracts, I have been able to do that, and I have enjoyed making a contribution to something bigger (e.g. a larger project). I'm pleased I haven't been running the projects but being able to provide input from my corner of the universe has been a significant win for me.

3. Collaboration. Working with people has been a great win for me too. Some of the people I've worked with have known I had survived a stroke and others haven't. My recovery has been strong and I know that from my looks and written word alone, people could not tell that I was recovering from a brain haemorrhage from less than a year ago. When I first started to work on the contracts and had to meet online with others in the team to discuss specific areas or topics I initially felt slightly apprehensive, but once I got stuck in, all that sense of anxiety went. I am a big believer in facing fears to eradicate them and this is another example. I love the popular meaning given to fear, False Evidence Appearing Real...and I also resonate with the concept of "walking up to" the fear and facing it head-on. Fear then dissolves instantly when that happens and all anxiety about what the mind 'thinks' will happen is proved to be nothing but BS.

Transformation Key: Look for the wins in everything that happens for you. Sometimes they will be obvious, and sometimes they may be hidden, but somewhere, they are there.

101

❧

11 February 2022: 6 Months? Nope 5

6 months? Nope, 5.

So I realised today that it is exactly 5 months to the date since the stroke!

For some reason, I had thought that it would be 6 months on Feb 11, but no it's 5 months.

Even though I say myself, that is incredible as my recovery progression is so strong.

Many within the world of stroke comment to me saying that my recovery is amazing.

Personally, others may take an opposing view, but I believe that my belief in the power of Source Energy/God/The Universe/Divine Intelligence/Universal Intelligence combined with my daily routines and determination balanced with gratitude,

> yoga, meditation and strength training has carried me through this journey (and still does to this very day).
>
> It never stops and never will stop.
>
> The practices I've developed will continue for my life! Claire does an amazing job of pushing me, I push myself too and Claire's incredible intuitive and emotional healing helps me so much. This is not an easy journey but the techniques she has taught me and that I've applied have worked wonders and like miracles.
>
> I'm excited for the future like never before. Every little thing in my life now carries a new sense of wonderment.

Leading up to this particular date (Feb 11, 2022), I was convinced that I was approaching 6 months since the stroke. It was only when the date actually arrived, I realised that it wasn't 6 months, but actually 5 months! Wow, I was jumping for joy inside, it was like another surprise birthday present that is literally like the 'icing on the cake' or ' the cherry on top'. Needless to say, I was very happy and it was a testament to all of the work I had been doing.

As well as the outer physical work, I had done so much inner work with Claire's guidance. I have to say that without the inner work, the outer work is worth shit. Both have to go hand-in-hand. I truly believe (and this was certainly the case for me) that too many people rely on only the outer work to fix their problems, but in my opinion, I don't believe that is truly effective.

I believe in the fundamental philosophy and understanding

that our thoughts create our reality. Everything happens in the meta-physical before we get to experience it in the physical. Some people may say that's woo-woo bullshit, and that's ok, they can say whatever they want, I'm totally cool with being a nut job if that's what people want to think. As I write this, I realise that this is the new me speaking my truth. It's so freeing to be able to speak one's truth without fear of judgement....I mean who the fuck are they to judge anyway?

So, back to inner and outer work. Everything in life is a balancing act. The yin and yang of transformation/healing/ recovery/growth/ expansion are always both inner and our work. We are conditioned to believe that it's all a matter of outer/physical work but that's not really effective. To truly experience the transformation, or the healing, or the recovery, or the growth and expansion, the physical work must be accompanied by inner work. By inner work, I mean emotional healing, listening to your inner God-self, and learning to ignore the fear-based ego voice that constantly wants to protect us by keeping us small. This inner work sounds easy but it's far from easy. In fact, it's as difficult as training for and running a marathon. The inner work means understanding your emotions and feelings. But remember, we have to accompany the inner work with the aligned outer work. So for me and my recovery, the outer work includes the discipline to exercise and doing physiotherapy; it means eating the right nutrition; it means listening to music that supports my recovery and so on. For other people and in other cases, the outer work is aligned action. In short, aligned action is taking action that aligns with positive feelings and the state of flow. Whenever the action is dis-aligned there is a build-up of resistance which does not serve the intended outcome.

On some days all of this work can get really tiresome so it's important to incorporate rest and play, but even activities of rest and play should be done with intention and on purpose. We are ALWAYS creating with our thoughts, it never ever stops whilst we are living and breathing. Many people are so careless with their thoughts. They will spend a short time focused and setting intentions to create the outcome they seek and then immediately default back to thoughts based on fear, doubt and unworthiness. When this happens all of the momentum established by the thoughts based on the target outcome are negated by the stronger and more dominant thought in the opposite direction. The result of this is that a lot of people remain stuck or progressively get worse results in their lives.

Transformation Key: All transformation/healing/recovery/ growth is achieved through a balance of inner and outer work.

102

13 February 2022: 5 Months Later

5 months later

As I got up this morning I thought to myself, "So, here we are 5 months after my body decided that it would throw me the biggest curve ball in my entire life (the brain haemorrhage) and how do I feel today?"

I decided to write this post as a means of recording this as a memory to look back on in the future.

This journey has been life-changing. "No shit Sherlock!", I laugh to myself as I think about that phrase, "Life changing. ". Yep, there's absolutely no doubt about that. Imagine your life as it is and turn the entire thing on its head! Hard to imagine isn't it?

If someone had said to me a year ago that I would be writing this post I would have dismissed it as almost nonsense. But of course, one never knows what's around the corner. My biggest advice to anyone is CYA. Cover Your Ass! If I had known what was coming I would have taken out an insurance plan with critical illness cover to take away the financial worry.

I am sitting here in my latest car as I write this. Even the cars have changed. We had to sell our VW Transporter and now I drive a go-cart!! Well not quite a go-cart but the Peugeot 107 is actually like a go-cart...and actually I love it; it's great fun; it's OLEZ compliant, £20 tax per year, returns high MPG and it's great fun to drive. I have ideas to boy-racer it. I don't give a crap what others might think about my ideas to boy-racer it. Loud exhaust, tailgate spoiler, alloy wheels....the whole deal...yes!! Love love love it!! Anyway, it's not like that today and I still love it anyway....But I have big ideas!!I've driven my son to rugby this morning and I'm sat here waiting for kick-off in the car (go-cart) in the pouring rain feeling utterly grateful although the rain could bugger off if it wanted (that would be better).

So, 5 months later...what's it like?

Everything has changed.

My brain is recovering from brain damage.

My physical abilities were totally impaired but I'm overcoming the (now constant) feeling of falling. It used to be dizziness and nausea but now it's a falling feeling but I can overcome that as well....that will change to something else soon and eventually full stability will return. I now do yoga twice a day along with 50 press-ups morning and night. I'm determined to get my strength back to what it was (3 months of almost nothing took *its toll on my body strength).*

I haven't worked full-time in 5 months and can't see myself doing so for a long time. In fact, the stress associated with full-time work does not appeal in the slightest. I do bits of creative marketing writing for customers which I enjoy as it capitalises on my 30+ years in customer experience and SaaS software and my writing skills. I still support individuals in a team of almost 100 members in my forex and crypto biz. I learn and teach about the metaverse space (NFTs, DeFi, Gaming etc.)...I find the future world fascinating and full of opportunities. I love writing. I love candle making. I sometimes wonder, what is going to actually make me decent money? I have no idea of that answer but I'm learning to embrace the unknown as best I can. My life has become richer in many ways that I could not have predicted, but financial stability would be nice.I find I have huge empathy for those with brain injury, either from stroke or other illnesses. Nothing can prepare one for brain damage, it's like nothing else I've ever experienced. The feeling of being isolated in one's own head is not nice. Because I generally look ok and because I generally navigate my way around the world (e.g. driving, walking the dog, shopping, going to my son's rugby etc.), I think people think I'm ok, but actually I'm not. The anxiety is quite acute. I'm sure that will pass as my confidence in all aspects of life gets better and better.

Confusion and memory. If I get confused by the smallest of things I get upset (well, my brain does). If I've been told we're doing one thing and then that changes to something else, my brain goes into a storm. Imagine a lightning storm in your head and you'll get an idea of the type of confusion that is taking place. It's not nice and has an impact on my confidence which then leads to anxiety etc. If we have a plan let's please stick to it or if it's changed let's make the communication really clear, then my brain can adjust ok. Memory. Some things I just instantly forget and yet other things go in forever. I haven't yet found a pattern to this. I remember the most complex of subjects and then forget the simplest of things...sometimes! On another occasion, it might be the complete reverse. As I say, there is no pattern on this one. If I've forgotten, I've forgotten, there's nothing I can do about that, I just apologise and ask for a reminder.

I use an App called Lumosity for brain training, it's brilliant, and my scores are getting better and better so I'm confident that my confusion and memory will get better over time.

So there we are. 5 months on and that is what life is like. I haven't covered it all but it's a decent record for me to look back on in the future.

Ok, the rain has eased, it's time to get a coffee and watch some rugby.

As I said in this post, if someone had said to me a year earlier that I would be writing that post, I would have completely dismissed the thought as utter nonsense, and yet there it is, February 13, 2022, and I'm writing about aspects of my life 5 months after a brain haemorrhage. Life is so frail. It could have been game over for me. My only prior experience of brain haemorrhage was in my childhood when the

30-something-year-old guy who lived in the same village was rushed into hospital one night and he was never seen again!

I had survived. It wasn't game over for me. It was a complete rebirth and reboot of my life with all of the existing aspects still surrounding me like my relationships, my family, my kids and of course the love of my life, Claire. I recall Claire saying to me that it didn't matter if she had to push me around in a wheelchair for the rest of my life, she knew when I was in the hospital that I was still in there despite not being able to walk and function fully. That is when you know that you're with your love for life. Claire has been a rock to me and even though there was a period during which I had to face my demons alone, she was still there helping me and guiding me.

It was fitting that during a weekend visit to Norwich in June 2022 when Claire was attending a workshop I had the opportunity to spend time alone (with Toby dog of course). I took myself off on the Saturday to explore the Norfolk and Suffolk coastline with Toby. As I walked a stretch of beach I let the voice of God / Higher Self / Higher Consciousness speak to me and guide me. Eventually, I stopped to rest, ate some lunch, drank some water and then wrote this:

"I used to hear one dominant voice in my head. It was relentless and it had no mercy. It was fuelled by fear and it had a purpose to cause worry and doubt within me. I would feel lost because I knew there was a rest bite to be found somewhere deep in my soul but it remained hidden. I used to feel an overwhelming sadness but the welcome relief from tears would never happen. It was like torture.

On and on, year after year the same perpetual grip of unhappiness. Why would the voice of fear never go away?

After the brain trauma of the haemorrhage and stroke on Sept 11, 2021 (exactly 9 months ago), I had no option but to stop and re-boot my entire life. Precious elements remained, like my family and fiancé Claire and the beautiful surroundings and home in which we lived, but I, my whole self, had an opportunity to transform and I metaphorically grasped the opportunity with open arms

In that transformation, I found the glory of a new voice. A voice of kindness, peace and love. I would say I discovered the voice of God within me. I say discovered, I feel I should say I rediscovered because the voice of God is in everyone and we were born with it fully speaking to us but we then become conditioned into silencing that voice and replacing it with something fear-based.

Today as I walk alone with Toby dog on a beautiful Norfolk beach, I get to hear that voice again. In silence, except for the wind and waves, I can listen to a voice that leaves clues in the form of intuitive nudges and pulls to go here, walk there, stop here, take that picture, now that one and why? Because of this very message. The message that effortlessly pours out of me in my writing after I've stopped to sit back at a spot where I photographed poppies on the shore.

I called this rediscovery "The Gift". Claire always said to me that I would find a gift from the stroke. I think I just have."

It took a further 4 months from the post in February at the rugby club to then find "the gift" and I think "the gift" is in actual fact multiple gifts but without doubt the biggest of all those gifts is my rediscovered ability to be able to hear the voice of my god-self. Each and every one of us has that voice within us. Unfortunately, for many of us, the voice cannot be heard because of all the noise, chatter, bullshit and distractions in our lives. We are bombarded with all this other 'stuff' that drowns out our God-self voice until we have those moments alone or we witness a beautiful sunset or dawn, or feel the sea between our toes, or marvel at the natural beauty of...(take your pick, God is everywhere). I use the word, God, not in any religious sense but as a simple way to represent universal consciousness or divine intelligence, and I mean the kind of intelligence that originally set the universe in motion, a universal consciousness that first imagined a big bang out of pure nothingness (the void), an intelligence that you and I possess through our creative imaginations and we feel in our hearts, and an intelligence that has the ability to heal and create miracles when allowed to do so.

This gift and knowing is my transformation. In that way, I suppose it is very personal but in the name of giving, my intention is that you too can learn from this experience so it becomes the gift that keeps on giving. It is your gift too.

Transformation Key: Find silence and stillness in your life and you will start to hear your God-self.

103

13 February, 2022:
Sending Love

Sending love.

As I did my yoga and strength exercises tonight I had an overwhelming feeling of love wash over me.

I felt a love and peace like never before; so much so that I was moved to send my love to anyone:

Who feels frightened

Who feels lonely

Who feels confused

Who feels rejected

Who feels weakness

If this applies to you then please feel and accept this love that I was blessed with tonight. It's a simple but effective gift.

If this does not apply to you then feel and accept this love to you

anyway and pass it on as there's always plenty to go around.
#love

People say that time is a healer, but time is a human-made construct designed to help us navigate the world. The true healer is love.

This is not the love from an external source (e.g. your dog), or another human being (e.g. your spouse, partner or lover), I am referring to the love that is within and all around. I am referring to a love that is the source of the spiritual universe and from which all things arise. This is the love of divine consciousness. This is a love that you feel in your heart regardless of external circumstances. I would say, this is the love from which all things are made.

This love is the true source of all healing and transformation.

Unfortunately, I had to experience an almost fatal event before I truly understood this. I had read this type of thing numerous times before and "understood" it intellectually, but if I'm honest with myself, I hadn't fully embodied it.

People call these types of change your "Come to Jesus moment", but when it actually occurs it is so utterly deep and profound that it almost cannot be described in the written word. And I don't mean come to Jesus in the Christian religious sense, it is a more a Christ consciousness sense or a Buddha sense rather than Buddhist religion. I am not against any religion and I don't advocate one religion over another, but I am referring to a deeper and more wider understanding of a God that spans all religions and faiths described by humans. My faith is based on Quantum Physics and pure divine Love rather than a religious-based doctrine and set of rules.

When I think back to my childhood and former pre-stroke days, I always had a deep feeling and knowing that we are all God. I can imagine the reaction of any religious leader accusing me of heresy because this kind of thinking goes against any religious doctrine. But the irony is that I love all religions for the universal foundational connection with God. What I don't subscribe to is any one religion having more validity over another. So many wars have been fought throughout the ages in the name of God and actually, they've always been about ego power and control and nothing to do with God and true divine love.

I digressed, but I think it's an important distinction that I needed to make clear.

When I truly felt the love of God inside of me, I knew I had re-found myself and my true essence and that essence is love.

Do I have love for everyone and all things? Well actually yes. Even those that have wronged me and still upset me to this day. I realise that if I get upset it is because the upset (e.g. anger, bitterness, frustration, sadness, etc.) resides in me and the person just happens to be the trigger of those emotions in me. Therefore the work that I need to do, and continue to do every time it occurs, is to release the emotion that is held or stuck within me. The process of releasing the emotion results in a feeling of love. Think of it this way... when the 'negative' emotion is released from my body, rather than leaving an empty void, the emptiness is immediately replaced by love. I think that's amazing. There's no having to go to the Love Station (think Gas Station) to fill up the empty tank with love. The love just floods in automatically... now that is the abundance of divine love that we all have unlimited access to if we choose. Wow, what a gift!

Transformation Key: If something or someone is triggering an unwanted emotion within you. Do the work to release that emotion and it will be immediately replaced by the unlimited supply of divine love.

104

14 February, 2022: Date Night

Date night

OMG, I've never enjoyed the experience of cinema quite so much as tonight.

Beautiful Claire organised tickets (thanks Gemma) and we went to watch "Marry Me".

It was in proper chic flic romantic comedy territory but I loved it ...mind you, with Jennifer Lopez playing a starring role it certainly helped a bit, I can't lie.

On our way home we stopped and looked up at the stars through the panoramic sunroof in our other new car - a 9-year-old Nissan Quasqai + 2...fully loaded with all the goodies.

It was a lush evening and a lush moment. As I looked up at the stars and moon through the sunroof I was brought to tears with

> *sheer gratitude for the moment...these thoughts passed through*
> *my mind:*
> *I am really alive*
> *I am recovering*
> *This moment is happening*
> *The stars and moon look incredible*
> *I'm sharing this moment with the love of my life*
>
> *I want to breathe it all in and savour every part of it all*
> *Life is beautiful*
> *Happy Valentine*
>
> *Love to all*

To feel alive once more and experience a typical human "date night" again with Claire was pure magic.

For most people going to the cinema and watching a movie is kind of "normal" I guess. It's something we can take for granted without much thought beyond enjoying the movie (hopefully) and perhaps eating a few snacks. Typically, we decide what we want to see, we book the tickets, rock up to the movie theatre/cinema, enjoy the art of the movie and then head back home hopefully feeling contented and satisfied.

For me, it was like going to the movies for the very first time and then after we left and Claire drove the car home we stopped and rolled the seats into the laying position and looked up at the stars through the panoramic roof of the car.

It was a cold, clear night but the car was warm enough to retain heat for about 5 mins comfortably. As we lay there looking up at the stars on that cold night, I had to take a moment to breathe it all in.

These kinds of moments happen a lot more since the stroke and they are another aspect of "The Gift", and they are magical.

There are moments when the world seems to stand still and I get to experience life in almost slow-motion. In the slow-motion version of reality, the idea of reality made up of a series of images comes into play. Imagine every aspect of reality being played on a movie screen and then slowed to the point where each frame is depicted in its original form. It probably sounds like I'm mad, but I don't actually see these 'frames' because my brain and mind cannot operate at that intense speed to actually detect that, but in my imagination, it can get a sense of it. Pre-stroke I had never perceived reality like that but I suppose by perceiving reality as a series of frames in a movie that means that the movie can be edited. That means that life can be edited and changed.

When perceiving reality in this "movie" frame-by-frame way, and when considering any desired change or transformation of one's life or circumstances, the question becomes, what form of editing needs to occur? So if we decide to change our life we would have to edit not just one frame of the movie but literally hundreds or thousands or hundreds of thousands. If we thought that changing just one frame would make a difference, it wouldn't, the altered frame would just become a blur in an otherwise pre-defined movie.

As I lay there looking up at the stars and observing the cosmos in the night sky above my head, these thoughts would run through my head and it was a moment when everything started to make sense. It was yet more evidence of how another spark of magic had been bestowed upon me. I am alive, I am recovering, I am here, I am all that I am.

Transformation Key: If you want to make a change in your life, you have the opportunity at any moment to start. How about starting now?

105

17 February, 2022: Talking To Me

> *Talking to me*
>
> *Today on my walk, I looked out at the view and I said to myself,*
> *"Hey God, talk to me please"...*
>
> *...and I heard the music playing in my coat pocket, I heard and*
> *felt the wind in my face, I sensed the warmth of the sun on my*
> *back, I smelt the farm in the distance, and then I heard the sky-*
> *larks as they chirped while establishing their nests in the field.*
>
> *"Thank you", I said, "I hear you, I feel you, I know you're with*
> *me and life is good."*
>
> *That is all*
>
> *Namaste*

As my connection with God deepened I started to have more

conversations and would become aware of the presence of divine consciousness literally everywhere.

In everything, in everybody, and everywhere.

As this was a newfound ability to talk to God, I would play around with it. I suppose at some level there were moments when I would think that I was having a conversation or asking a question of a God outside of myself, but as time went on I realised that I was having the conversation in my head, it was all thoughts and I would hear a spoken response in my own voice. But it was apparent that the answers would also come from everything around me, not just my own voice in my head.

As I listened to music playing or looked at the trees, or listened to the birds, or the sound of the wind, felt the warmth of the late winter sun on my face, smelt the aroma of cows from the farm in the distance, all of it was magical, all of it was divine consciousness (God) and all of it was forming the reality that I made of it.

I was shifting from surviving a stroke to a new sense of thriving. Of course, materially, we were still surviving rather than thriving, but at the spiritual level, I had never felt so good. I was definitely on the up!

Transformation Key: See the potentiality in all moments and all things. Divine consciousness is everywhere and in all things in every moment. Relish in the exquisiteness of life.

106

18 February, 2022: Writing

Writing

For the past two days, I've buried myself in my writing.

I'm writing a book documenting my personal journey of a brain haemorrhage (stroke), my recovery and survival, and my path to redemption.

The recovery and redemption are still a work in progress and in many ways will always be ongoing forever.

I've written about 5000 words so far and there's so much more to do.

I've had some brilliant advice from Sue Stone for which I am so grateful (thanks Sue) and others have connected me with some incredible resources and I'm excited to see how that all unfolds.

In the meantime, here's a very short extract from the period when I initially became aware of the journey of recovery that I was about to embark upon...

"..I realised early in my recovery that achieving goals might take me some time and I accepted that, but determination was a hallmark of my character that seemed to show itself when I needed it, and this was one of those moments.Equally, alongside determination, I'd say that other overriding aspects of my recovery have been, and still are, surrender and acceptance. There are many words that come to mind: resilience, fortitude, determination, strength, along with surrender, acceptance, forgiveness, grace, and the most powerful word of all is love.

Self-love (or self-care) has played a very important part in my recovery. I mean this primarily in the mental and emotional sense and I truly believe that my spirituality and faith in a higher intelligence (God is an ok word if you want) has contributed greatly to my discovery of peace throughout my recovery from this life-changing stroke."

More to come... Stay tuned!

So it was happening, this book was well underway. 5000 words at the time of that post in Feb 2022 and now here I am on 23 Aug 2022, some 6 months later, and the word count says 76,192! Wow, I can't actually believe it, and just 16,705 of those words are from the posts. That means that about 60k words are from the additional narrative that pours through me.

It's quite incredible how this process of writing has been so cathartic and emotional. I write while one of my favourite playlists plays in my headphones, so I am immersed in the writing experience to allow all the memories and feelings to flow through me. I think most of the writing has been 'channelled' through me from divine consciousness and I have been able to call upon my experiences following each post as I write the additional narrative.

At this point, as I write I have no idea where or what this book will lead to, but that is ok. I have visions and ideas which shall remain in my heart and as they unfold I shall smile and thank my God-self for each physical manifestation as and when it occurs.

I have no idea when the effects of the stroke will finally leave me but I have a sense that one day I will wake up and notice that a symptom (or strangeness) that I have become accustomed to will have gone. Perhaps, some symptoms will remain with me for the rest of my life, but I'm okay with that, I am so utterly and profoundly grateful to be alive and have the opportunity to 'do life' in a whole new way with a deeper connection to God within me.

My relationship with God and the divine consciousness in everything will continue for the rest of my life. I know that deep in my soul. It will be a continual unfolding of knowing and understanding that will always delight me in every new knowing, in every new layer of awareness and practice. This is it, no turning back now, not now, this is beautiful!

Transformation Key: The relationship within yourself to divine consciousness is a continuous journey, it is never done. Enjoy the journey in all its glory.

107

19 February 2022: It's Not All Rainbows and Unicorns

it's not all rainbows and unicorns, some days it actually feels pretty crappy and sad.

...and that is ok... feeling crappy and sad is allowed.

I felt that this morning. I felt crappy and sad because I'm tired of feeling like I'm drunk for 5+ months. Some people respond jokingly with that it must be great or something similar. I understand and I don't judge anyone for that response. But quite frankly, it's really not great at all. Feeling drunk pretty much all the time (except when I'm driving, writing or sleeping) is debilitating and frustrating. Luckily, and through sheer determination, I haven't ever fallen over! I've also mastered some tricky yoga poses that push my balance to the max (still have not fallen over) so I'm coping ok. Today (or that moment) was just a crappy moment, and that's ok they happen and they mean nothing.

I cannot wait for the day when the feeling has stopped. I know that one day that will be the case and I will celebrate hard.

I said to Claire that it would be like winning the lottery!

My advice today is twofold:

1. *If you're having a crappy, sad day and you want to cry then cry. It's ok. Let the emotion through so that it doesn't become stuck in your body. Much better out than in. Don't judge yourself for the sadness, just witness it and nothing more.*

2. *If you're fortunate to have a healthy brain then try to be grateful for your own incredible abilities for you have already won the lottery. You are already blessed with rainbows and unicorns*

With love

Well it couldn't be all plain sailing, could it? My recovery was going strong. My connection with God within me was out of this world. Massive spiritual awakenings in moment after moment. It was going well right?

But there are still moments within our lives when we feel sad, but the problem we humans have is we like to make a story out of the sadness and we have this obsession with giving the emotion (e.g. sadness) some form of meaning, which is actually pointless. It's much better to just feel the emotion (like sadness) and let the accompanying tears just flow for no other reason than just letting them flow. I have to give the credit to Claire for this insight and modality, and there are times when I think I've mastered it and then a situation occurs that trips me up and she (mostly gently) reminds me of this strategy. I call it a highly advanced emotional intelligence. She should bottle it and sell it; she would make a fortune!

At first, this is hard to do because we want to get wrapped up in a story. "I'm upset because..." Forget it! That just reinforces the power of the story and that just serves to make the situation worse. This may sound like I'm unsympathetic, but actually, it is the reverse. I have the deepest sympathy for anyone who is desperately sad, I mean for fucks sake, I've been there, got the shitty t-shirt and a whole lot more, but I can tell you from first-hand experience the way to navigate these tough times is to adopt this 'let it out' strategy. If it's anger, then find a punch bag, if it's sadness, cry, if it's frustration then scream into the pillow. Don't take your emotions out on anyone else because that is just not fair on them. It's hard not to project onto someone else, but even if you are the centre of your drama (which you always are), remember that other people are navigating their own lives too. So give yourself and those around you a break and deal with your emotions. I know it's hard but you can do it and by doing so you will become empowered.

Transformation Key: Learn the power of advanced emotional intelligence. It is the most empowering, life-changing tool you will ever possess.

108

❦

22 February, 2022:
Powering Recovery

Powering recovery.

I have to say that sometimes I blow my own mind.

When I considered the massive imbalance that affected my body just 5+ months ok, I'm shocked that today I am able to walk across Dartmoor in high winds.

If someone had said I'd be doing this when I took my first tentative steps in hospital 1 week after the brain haemorrhage that turned my life entirely on its head, I would have said, "Not a chance!!"

This kind of recovery takes many things:

Luck - yes, the 4cm bleed in my cerebellum could have caused so much more damage than it did, but I was lucky and the damage was minimal (I can't find another suitable word).

Determination - every day I have to do the work; the work of physiotherapy; the work of strength training; the work of yoga. I am fortunate that I enjoy physical exercise so I find the ability to motivate myself fairly easy.

Grace - As I've undertaken the exercises and work I've had to give myself plenty of grace and forgiveness when I've found the work too hard or the stretch just too far. So the outcome at this moment (on this day) is that I am able to walk and climb some of the Tors of Dartmoor. To a non-stroke survivor, this might be a normal activity but to me this aspect of my journey of recovery is amazing!!

I'm so bloody chuffed!!!

It was so windy on Dartmoor! For those unfamiliar with Dartmoor, it is an area of outstanding natural beauty in Devon, in the southwest of England. It is a vast area of open ground; it's windy, it's desolate and it can be very bleak, indeed. It's not a place to go in the middle of winter or a place to go wondering during bad weather. It's a dangerous place. It's a place where the British armed forces train their troops for outdoor survival.

Claire had booked a beautiful cottage for us to stay in, which was right on the edge of Dartmoor and we spent the few days we were there exploring the Tors within the area. Tors are outcrops of rock in high areas of Dartmoor. To walk to a Tor often involves a fairly steep climb and walking across the open, windy moorland.

It was insanely windy when we visited but it was exhilarating to feel the strength of the wind and find shelter within the rocks. Luckily it didn't rain or else I think we would have swiftly abandoned our Tor adventures as that would have been horrible.

As it was only February the light of the day would still fade by late afternoon and before dark we would head home to our beautiful cottage to make a family dinner, light the fire and watch a movie or play a game. I recall that one morning it rained so another Tor adventure would have to wait until the rain had stopped. We decided to play Cluedo. I hadn't played Cluedo since I was a child. It was great fun and all the children, Claire and I really enjoyed it. Before we knew it, the rain had stopped, the fire had gone out and we were planning our next exploring adventure on Dartmoor. It was a lovely break for all the family.

Transformation Key: Allow adventure to enter your life as it can open up new experiences. Life is for living.

109

$\approx$

26 February, 2022:
Incremental Change

Incremental Change.

I've seen a lot of rhetoric about how incremental change is not necessarily the source of overall transformation...I disagree.

In my own recovery from the brain injury caused by a brain haemorrhage (stroke) which occurred almost 6 months ago, I am living proof of the benefit of small incremental changes.

I am pleased to say that my own recovery and improvements in my mental, physical, emotional and spiritual well-being have all been attributed to tiny incremental improvements that have taken place all along this journey over the past 6 months (and it's continuing).

There are many days when the improvements are not that noticeable or I might struggle (physically, mentally, emotionally or spiritually). Hey I'm human after all and as a human, I want instant gratification the same as the next person, but in the recovery game, instant results are not a reasonable expectation.

Do we put unreasonable expectations on others and ourselves? Perhaps so.

Had I tried to walk and access my phone just a few months ago then I would have felt dizzy and I wouldn't have been capable. Yesterday, I did this seemingly simple task. Having experienced brain injury I can assure you this is not easy. The complex signalling and muscle coordination that the brain is controlling is out of this world. It is my determination and grace, along with my focus on doing the work when I want to quit, that has culminated in this remarkable rebuild that enables these results. So I make the case with living evidence that slow, strong and steady does work, it may not be the sexy way but it does work!!!

Have a great day

Some transformations might be instant whilst others may take time to occur. In my experience of my brain recovery, the process was both fast and slow. What do I mean by that? When I consider that just 5 months before this post of 26 February 2022, I was unable to walk and the disorientation and dizziness that I was experiencing made me horribly nauseous. Equally, 5 months was crazy fast too. I had persevered to do the exercises when I didn't want to. I had pushed myself gracefully to do the extra stretch, the extra step, the extra head turn. I had found the strength within me to keep going and push just a little further than I had wanted. I had navigated the dark depth of depression. I had started to heal long-held emotional wounds from years previous. I had gone to hell and back and got the T-shirt, all in 5 months. Simultaneously when I looked at or considered each moment or day at a time, it seemed like a lifetime, so slow.

The huge lesson from this is that perseverance, determination, acceptance, surrender, grace and forgiveness all play a vital role in maintaining a steady path to a recovery that is strong.

To this very day, I still feel the effects of the injury to my brain, but once again, through all the qualities listed above, each day my confidence to live with the effects grows stronger all the time. I am now sailing and I recently used a Stand Up Paddle-board (SUP) for the very first time in my life.

As I write this and mention the SUP, it is still less than 12 months since the stroke. I cannot imagine what the physio team in the hospital, the same people who had first helped me take those "Bambi-like" steps, would make of the news that less than a year later the very same bloke was seen on the sea and on a lake balancing and paddling a SUP! Mad some might say, but this shows what is possible with the right mindset, determination, acceptance, surrender and grace.

Transformation Key: Anything is possible with the right mindset, determination, acceptance, surrender and grace. Anyone is capable of anything.

110

28 February, 2022: Milestones

Milestones.

It's all about milestones right? Well maybe it is, I don't know for sure.

But what I do know is today as I write this book, I've crossed the milestone of 15000 words.

As I recall the memories and moments from the stroke and the journey of recovery I find the process very cathartic. I laugh; I cry; I feel the feels; I witness the emotions, and I type as the words pour through me.

I knew posts like this would serve to help tell the story. In the story, I've just reached early October 2021 so there is a vast journey still to tell so I cannot foresee how many words this will be in total (I estimate 30k at least).

> *But the number of words doesn't really matter; it's the message of awareness and transformation taking place within the words that really matter.*
>
> *I've become and am becoming a new version of me. Me v3 it's the version in the book. I wrote today that the stroke was a gift. I never thought I'd say that but in the moment of connected writing it's amazing what gets channelled through; I'm just the messenger after all.*

This book was starting to take shape. It hasn't been a sprint but a marathon. In terms of time, I have not spent much time during the working day because of, guess what, working!

The contracts that I secured have been occupying my time. But whenever I have a free evening I have been writing this book. I wasn't entirely sure how it would take shape and what would even constitute some kind of end but that is now very clear to me and no, we're not there yet!

I've taken my laptop to the rugby club when my son has been to gym-based strength and conditioning training in the summer months.

I've taken every opportunity I've had outside of my work contracts to write this book. It's been an amazing journey that has allowed me to re-live the entire experience again and release all the traumatic emotions associated with the brain haemorrhage, the journey of recovery, whilst also celebrating those moments of the spiritual journey of deeper transformation than I could have ever imagined. Many people say that re-living trauma is not good but I would take a different view. Re-living the experience has helped me tremendously, but it's been a repeat over a long period and I've shed many tears in the process of writing, but the results have been remarkable.

The process of writing has also led to so many new revelations. First and foremost, I love writing. If I could become a full-time author then I would be as happy as a pig in poo. Who knows what will come of this but as it stands today I fund this by working part-time on IT-based business contracts and that is great and I am eternally grateful to be able to do that.

Writing allows my connection with the divine consciousness (God) to flow through me. I fire up the laptop, find my favourite recovery playlist on my phone, stick on the Bluetooth headphones and that's it, I'm away, just totally lost in the writing and the flow of the words.

So at the end of February (as posted) I had written 15000 words and estimated this might go to 30000 words. As I write this, the word count in Pages states 78,908 words. Let's just say I'm rubbish at estimating. It's really not my best skill. So I've now given up trying to estimate how many words this book will be. The message within the words and the enjoyment of writing are the important factors in this project.

Transformation Key: There may be distractions along the

journey of transformation but stick at it and don't ever stop. Keep moving forward and don't give up.

III

⚜

4 March, 2022: Reading

> *Reading.*
>
> *I'm really looking forward to starting this later on...*
>
> *...and on the subject of books, I had a wonderful call with Nicky Marshall today discussing publishing and all of the amazing work that she has accomplished with her own publishing business since her own stroke 12 years ago. Really inspiring and insightful thank you, Nicky!!*
>
> *More book news to follow, stay tuned.*
>
> *The word count of my draft manuscript is now almost 23000!!*

When I saw this book listed on a very well-known online bookstore I had to order it! In my opinion, "One Truth, One Law: I am, I Create" by Erin Werley is a masterpiece.

All my life I have had this feeling that I am God. Ok, that

sounds crazy I know and I've mentioned before that I would be cast into the pits of hell by those religious sorts. But I don't mean that I am exclusively (just me) God. No, I believe every one of us is God.

Whoah, that's big, right? Yes, it's massive. It's not only massive as a statement, but it's also massive because of our incredible creative power. When I read this book, I couldn't believe it, there was someone else channelling and saying the exact same thing. What is so sad is that most of the human race appears to let themselves become trapped and conditioned by fear and the dominance of the ego-mind and so they create a life for themselves they do not want. Most of us are guilty of switching off, dumbing down and ignoring this massive creative ability.

Did you know that we create our reality in the mind? We construct it all in the mind. Our senses help us navigate the 3D earth, but we have so many more senses that many of us just ignore. We are spiritual beings having a human experience. We are energy. I've always believed this and in a deeper part of me, I've always known this. This is why I am not afraid of death. I just consider death as passing from this earthly realm back to pure source energy, so in that sense is it death at all? It's just another form of transformation. Transformation (or change) is constant. We cannot stop it and fight it. Now that said, the human experience is wonderful.

When I had come close to transforming back to pure source energy I woke up! I woke up to the magic of this earthly realm. I had been asleep in a dream and my ego-mind was making my dream increasingly difficult and stressful until one day on September 11, 2021, I had created the ultimate experience for myself in the form of a brain haemorrhage.

You may ask, what did I just read? I created the brain haemorrhage? Yes, that's right. At some level, I created that experience. Nothing happened to me, it was always for me. And remember me (and you) are forms of God.

On June 20, 2022, I wrote this note on my phone. It was a conversation with God (or should I say the drop of God within me):

Simon: So why did I have the brain haemorrhage?

God: Because I knew you wouldn't die. I knew you could handle it. I knew you were strong enough.

Simon: Is there a meaning to it?

God: Not really. I just wanted to experience the type of brain injury you experienced. Thank you.

Simon: Am I making a good recovery?

God: Yes, amazing and you are shining the light for others. You're giving people hope so keep going.

Simon: Is that why I have to write the book?

God: Yes, don't stop.

So there it is. God just wanted to experience it all. You see if God is pure source energy then God can only experience earthly experiences through us humans. Isn't that amazing? What this means is that if we have the power of God within us we can use that power for all manner of good things. I know that some people or even many people might think I've lost my marbles but I'm ok with that. I know that I am of sound mind as I write this, and that's good enough for me.

Let's get back to how amazing and mind-bogglingly powerful we are, in that we create our 3D reality within our brains. How do I know this? It's simple. When I experienced the brain haemorrhage my version of reality became completely disoriented. No one else experienced the same distortion. It was only me. I alone experienced that distortion. Everything shifted by 90 degrees; what was originally horizontal became vertical and vice-versa. My version of reality changed radically because my brain was in the process of being damaged. So that is how I know (for a fact) that we make up our own reality in our heads (our brains).

So, the next time you experience a beautiful sunset, the sound of the birds in the trees, the feel of the air on your face, the smell of the ocean spray... remind yourself just how amazing you are and feel the warmth in your heart rise through your body, for that is pure love in those moments. Those things are incredible so remember to congratulate yourself on just how amazing you are.

Transformation Key: You have the power of divine consciousness running through you at all times and you are brilliant in your humanness.

112

<!-- decorative ornament -->

7 March, 2022: Yoga

Yoga is a fundamental must-have in my recovery routine.

I've always loved a bit of flow in my daily routine but now it contributes so much to the strength and depth of my recovery and reboot as a new human.

This is the nighttime scene in our lounge before I head up to bed. I put on some amazing zen music (above and beyond flow state is a favourite) find a fake fireplace on YouTube and get into my flow.

Everything about this moment lights up my soul. It provides a perfect opportunity to give thanks for the day and send gratitude and love out into the world (I think we need that more than ever right now).

So namaste my friends (I see you, I honour you)

Yoga and making intentional time and space to strengthen

my body and deep breathing into various stretches has been a vital force in my recovery.

I like to vary the frequency so I don't get 'stuck in a rut' with my routine. I was doing a practice twice a day, every day. More recently through the summer months that has become once a day for 5 days a week. As we head back into the winter months I might steadily increase the frequency again. The reason for easing off in the summer is that my general mental well-being is better in the summer than in the winter, so I use the more frequent routine to help me navigate the winter blues as well as help my strength, brain recovery and connection with the divine.

I've mentioned before that I combine yoga, pilates and strength training within a series of flows. I do this whilst listening to the same playlist as when I'm walking around the woods and when I'm writing this book.

So what is this playlist? I've been a fan of streaming music services for years and on the one beginning with 'S' I discovered a playlist called Musical Therapy. It is primarily gentle piano-based with no beat and no vocals. Each track is very emotive and it has helped throughout my recovery. In fact, it could be said that the playlist has been the soundtrack to my recovery, spiritual awakening and transformation. I have created my own playlist called "The Gift" to accompany this book.

Transformation Key: Let the combination of gentle soothing music and yoga calm your mind and help you build the inner strength for transformation.

113

⚜

8 March, 2022: Fun All The Way

Fun All The Way.

I've owned numerous cars in the "nice" category such as BMW and Jaguar but this little car puts the biggest smile on my face. Far more than anything I've driven before.

With its tiny 1000 cc engine and basic levels of luxury (yep it has electric windows and air-con) it's perfect for me in this current period of my stroke recovery. All I want is to run the kids to school and do the grocery shopping....and this little car is perfect....and super economical too ◈ I've hooked up Bluetooth and can stream Anjunadeep and #ABGT as we zip around.

Don't get me wrong, I love the look of some of the modern models out there, there are so many stunning examples. But still, this little go-cart absolutely lights up my soul when I drive it.

> *I have big modification ideas for this and people will think I'm a 17-year-old boy racer, but I don't give a stuff what others think, nothing beats the fun I get from zipping around in this.*

I was referring to "Little Whizzy", a black Peugeot 107. Whizzy is great fun and all the kids are amazed at the space inside and the sense of flying along even at 45mph!

I've previously owned an array of other cars in my life and whilst some of them did have the luxury perks which was nice, there is something a little more raw about the driving experience of Whizzy. Some might say basic, but in all honesty, the air conditioning (and heating) is the best I've had in any car for years! She's great fun and so far, very reliable.

The only problem I've encountered is the sense that other road users think they can squeeze us out of the way, which is a little concerning sometimes I must say, so in recent months I've taken to adopting a driving approach similar to that of riding a motorcycle which is to drive with the headlights on. It seems to work and helps draw attention from other drivers that we are on the road ahead.

The other thing I've noticed is a feeling that other road users are driving very close behind. When you look at the size of the car, it's easy to see why. It's tiny. The boot space is almost non-existent with enough space for a few large bags of shopping.

So other than the limited luxury, lack of boot space and

the feeling that other users want to push me off the road, Little Whizzy is great fun and an amazing asset. Whizzy has enabled me to help with several driving trips and given me independence in my recovery. I drive myself to the doctor's surgery, pick up my medication prescription, drive the kids to and from school, go shopping when I'm not working, make visits to my family and run Claire out at the weekends or nights out.

Before I had the stroke, I always said that I didn't need to drive the Jaguar which I had owned since 2010. It was getting a bit tired and was looking like the ongoing maintenance costs to keep it would overtake the benefits of owning the car, so I had thought on many occasions that all I really needed was a cheap and economical run-around. That's exactly what I've got with Whizzy.

Once I'm finished with Whizzy and move on to something else, I hope that I will be able to pass it on to Charlotte as her first car.

Transformation Key: Don't ever look at something as being not good enough. Everything has value and worth.

114

13 March, 2022: Happy
Birthday My Love

Happy Birthday My Love.

Happy birthday Claire.

This has to be the most unusual birthday of yours ever!! It's been completely amazing that you have genuinely loved organising your own....everything!!! Presents, cake, table, balloons, literally everything.

I've felt completely useless but I've helped where I can. Others might judge me for that and I judge myself for that but you don't; you've never judged me; not ever and I cannot thank you enough for that.

I wish I had the capacity to do your birthday how I think you deserve (you deserve all the lovely things), but for now, I'll hand the entire day over to you knowing that one day I will (once

again) have the capacity to spoil you totally.
I love you baby - Happy birthday.

It was a strange feeling to let Claire organise her birthday. The ego-mind in me wanted to resist and say "No, but I must be the man and organise your birthday", but I could not think straight to organise Claire's birthday.

Planning Claire's birthday always used to stress me out even before having the stroke, but with the injured brain working hard to recover, the thought of trying to organise Claire's birthday to make it perfect was just not going to happen and for the first time I just let it all go and agreed with Claire that she could organise her own celebration.

Weirdly, she said it was brilliant and everything that she organised was like a surprise to her. Well, she certainly made it look like she enjoyed organising it all, anyway!

It was difficult for me to accept this at first but the relief I felt was huge. It made me realise just how much pressure I had put upon myself in previous years to make everything perfect, and I think on most occasions I had probably failed miserably in any case.

This characteristic of Claire is typical. She is a fantastic organiser, whereas I'm probably one of the worst, and I had always thought that I had to come up to her standard, which I couldn't possibly match. This time on Claire's 46th birthday,

I had to hoist the white flag of surrender and admit that I couldn't cope with the pressure.

One day, I will repay Claire for that self-organised birthday and everything else that she has done for me and I will make it up to her with something completely surprising and breathtaking. I love her so much and she is worthy of everything.

Transformation Key: It's ok to admit that you need help. Trying to push on when it feels wrong or stressful can do more harm than good. Go easy on yourself and let others help.

115

14 March, 2022: Face To Face

Face to Face.

Client conversations and introductions.

Super happy this morning to have had my first face-to-face intro meeting with a client (of a client) for over 6 months.

I cannot lie, I had a few nerves beforehand but I recognised that I was judging myself. With it being just a little over 6 months since the stroke had left me in a position of having to rebuild my injured brain, I have rebuilt (and I am still rebuilding) my physical well-being, my mental well-being, my emotional well-being, my social well-being and now another step towards my well-being from the perspective of value creation and earning a living. Today's intro call was a big deal for me.

I am forever grateful to Tim for his continued belief in my abilities despite my obvious life setback 6 months ago. His understanding and compassion to help me step back into the world of consultancy have been second to none. Thank you, Tim

As I reflect on the past six months of recovery I surprised myself at the pace of transformation. On Sept 14 2021 (6 months ago) I was barely alive and was starting a brain-rebuilding journey that I never ever would have considered was possible or would affect me in the first place (I mean what a total mind fuck!!!) and here I am on March 14, 2022, 6 months later, I'm having Teams calls with new clients again. Mind blown!!!!

Thank you to so many who have contributed to my recovery; the list is extensive, but thank you mostly to me and my brain for the tenacity, the belief and the vision to rebuild myself in double quick time.

The journey is not over (and perhaps it never will be tbh) but this feels like a huge milestone in this moment.

Don't ever doubt yourself or your abilities. As humans, we can do anything if we set out our intentions and channel our creative thoughts and actions accordingly.

Getting back into the world of work was a significant milestone. I was ready to jump back into the drive sitting but Tim, who provided me with the opportunity, understood that I would have my limitations and he didn't want to ask me to undertake work that would create stress or cause me to become fatigued.

The specific contract has been renewed twice with the client as the original time allocated was simply not sufficient. Stroke or no stroke, the task at hand was challenging. In fact, I found it interesting to observe behaviours in myself and others during the contract. When the contract started I found myself having to pick up from where someone else had worked before. Picking up from someone else is often difficult. We were dealing with a complex global enterprise IT scenario whereby the company were being sold to another parent company and the former parent company were no longer providing them with the IT services that they had become accustomed to. It probably sounds rather dull to someone not in that type of world, but this was the type of work that I had been involved with for years, and I soon got stuck in.

It was a complex situation and my part of the project was to help them understand which IT services they were going to be running in the future, which were outsourced, and so on. The term used is Service Catalogue (ok, ok, it does sound like it's a bit dull, yawn).

This sounds straightforward on the face of it, but there were so many different people and other organisations involved. At first, I had very little data to work with and it wasn't always clear to me what was actually wanted but then data started to come from multiple directions and I had to consume data in many formats into a structure that was consistent and would provide value.

Even as I write, the contract is still ongoing and it could

extend beyond the immediate requirement if the client can see the value in continuously improving their current state. We'll see...

I would say that being involved in this type of work has really boosted my confidence. I think it's understandable that I did question my confidence before starting the contract but I did feel ready and Tim reassured me that I could work at my own pace.

I wasn't sure whether Tim had said anything to the client about the stroke but I felt totally fine in the various Microsoft Teams-based meetings that I was involved with.

I recall that in a one-on-one meeting with the client, I asked her if she was aware of my history with the stroke. She said that yeah, Tim had mentioned something. We quickly moved on as if it was just a thing that happened and it was no big deal. This was the best way for me. I had come so far in my recovery that it almost wasn't a thing anymore. That is a significant milestone. Of course, the stroke happened, I'm not daft, but the fact that it doesn't define me now is really significant, and I believe that going back into a working environment helped with that shift in belief.

Transformation Key: Live as if the transformation has already happened and then it happens.

116

17 March 2022: The Relief and Gratitude Hit Me

The Relief and Gratitude Hit Me like a truck!!

As Claire and I walked out this morning I was overwhelmed by the huge sense of gratitude from the moment.

The moment of 6 months after the brain haemorrhage I am alive and I am re-engaging with customers, I am asking Claire if she'd like to take a break for the weekend, the moment of the early spring sun warming my face and the sound of the birds in the fields and hedgerows.....and so much more in my awareness...and all of it means so much more to me than it ever had before.

I cried and laughed simultaneously.

I am transformed and still transforming...wow what a journey this is...it is outstanding and the most amazing thing is the rejoicing in who I'm becoming (and I've become). I am an entirely

> *different man. I feel a continuous sense of peace and satisfac-*
> *tion...so much better than the old version. It is this realisation of*
> *this new version that invoked tears of relief, gratitude and joy.*
> *Wow*
> *With love*

As I grew stronger and more confident in my abilities it felt like I'd been given my life back again, but this time it was different. I was a more peaceful man, I had such gratitude for...well everything really, and this is still very much the case.

It is now almost 12 months after the stroke as it is late August 2022 as I write this. This post from March 2022 signified the immense gratitude I felt on that day. I am so pleased to say that the gratitude for the moment on any day has not dissi-pated. I have retained that peace and that deep appreciation for the gift of each moment in every day.

I enjoy life again. It is different. I am different. I still feel the effects of the brain injury. I stumble at times. When I stand or walk it still feels like I'm slightly drunk, but all that goes away in an instant if I drive, or I go sailing, or sit reading or writing. It's such an odd thing but if I stumble slightly or notice I've made a mistake with something, I just laugh to myself and don't make it mean that I'm broken or unable to function properly. Life is too short to be worried about stuff like that. Life is for living and enjoying myself and most of all I see that life is also about being true to myself. If I want to do something then I'll try to do it and, equally, if I don't want to do something, I won't. I have no intention of upsetting anyone but to live with truth and authenticity is one of the liberating things anyone can do.

When I reflect on this post from March, I remember the feeling of being completely overwhelmed with emotion as the relief and gratitude for my life washed over my body. It felt like I was basking in every aspect of my life and I was breathing in my life in that same moment. It's so hard to put into words and as I read this post from March, I am again so grateful that I had captured that memory in that moment so that I can look back and share these thoughts.

Transformation Key: Capture the moment and the memories so that you can celebrate your progress time and time again.

117

20 March, 2022: Bliss In The Forest

> *Bliss in the Forest.*
> *Good morning from a piece of paradise in Southern England.*

After I had suggested to Claire that we should go away somewhere, she found us a beautiful luxurious log cabin in Devon to stay.

It was perfection in every way. I remember on our first morning there, we woke up early and it was a clear crisp early Spring morning so we made our coffees and sat outside on the log cabin veranda. We were wrapped in thick cosy dressing gowns and sat on a swinging chair for two beneath heavy blankets. We stayed out there for a short while to breathe in the fresh morning air and listen to the sound of the birds in the crisp daylight of early spring before returning back inside to the warmth of a wonderful log fire in the burner.

We spent the weekend at the log cabin totally pampering ourselves with a log-fired hot tub and plenty of time for journaling, reading and walking. It was total bliss for Claire and I and it gave us time to acknowledge the journey we had been on together.

We took lovely food with us and the hosts of the log cabin provided a gorgeous welcome pack with plenty of tasty treats, however on the Sunday we booked ourselves a roast dinner lunch at a local pub. It was by far the best roast lunch dinner that both of us had ever enjoyed. It might have been the moment or it might have been the quality of the food but I can certainly confirm that the combination of it all created the perfect Sunday lunch.

We spent time walking together and exploring the immediate area surrounding the log cabin. Neither of us wanted to walk far but to be surrounded by such woodland beauty was beyond breathtaking.

The weekend and the log cabin were the perfect antithesis to the madness of the previous 6 months. Our family life was not completely 'out of the woods' but we had established a rhythm to our new version of life. I was coping better and better with my recovery and I was becoming a different man each and every day. Homeschooling included consistent help and support from a visiting teacher for our youngest child. We were making a consistent income that covered the expenses and allowed us to think about life's extras (like log cabin stays away) and my spiritual journey was unfolding for me.

Transformation Key: There are times when you can and should give yourself a break. Take the break and seize the moment for you deserve it.

118

⁘

25 March 2022: I Needed To Find Peace

I Needed To Find Peace

This week has been testing. We all have them right? Those times when so many things happen and life could easily get overwhelming.

I had set myself a plan to just walk today. I needed to find peace. I wanted to dedicate some intentional time to have a conversation with God (my kind and loving inner voice).

Walking alone allows me to find that peace and conversation and there's a number of places that hit the spot for me.

One such place is The Ridgeway, especially between Hackpen and Avebury. This is a place of ancient history and mysticism; of crop circles and stone circles; and today in springtime 2022, it is a place of the songs of nesting birds and the occasional batch of mountain bike riders. It is bliss in the mid-March sunshine as we approach the season of daylight savings (British Summer Time) here in the UK. It's a perfect spot to talk to God.

I recall 6 months ago (Sept 2021) when I was in hospital taking my first tentative steps after the stroke. I needed the arm and support of a physio nurse and I would look out of my window in hospital (Swindon GWH) and I would see The Ridgeway in the distance. "I'm going to get back and walk the Ridge", I said. My inner voice was setting out my future visions and getting me fuelled up. The journey of recovery never ends; it is a lifetime journey of continuous transformation. Moreover, life itself is a journey of continuous transformation...and wow what a journey!!!

With love from my inner voice.

I've always enjoyed the peace and solitude of walking alone. That's not to say I can't or don't want to walk with other people, but to me, being alone on a lovely walk allows my connection to my higher self and allows the God source within to come through. The voice of God within is peaceful and comforting. It is kind and calm and it fuels me with ideas and inspiration. When walking with others there is a tendency to chat with one another which is fine in itself, but it is impossible to have two conversations at once, I can't listen to God and someone else simultaneously.

I find it's possible to listen to my inner God voice in any setting within nature. I suppose each person will have their own preference but for me it is nature. Whether that's by spending time walking in the woods, sitting by a lake whilst the family is sailing or paddle boarding, or walking in special places with meaning or historical relevance.

On this particular occasion, it was the latter. I am lucky to live near a stretch of ancient road called The Ridgeway. It is littered with ancient burial sites, white horses carved into the hillsides and interspersed with ancient sites such as Avebury stone circle. As I walk along listening to my God voice, listening to the birds and the sound of the wind, I find myself lost in my thoughts of ancient humankind travelling to sites such as Avebury to celebrate the passing of time and the seasons, worshipping the sun and partaking in whatever kind of ritual was popular at that time.

Personally, I think it's important to try to find these types of time to be with yourself. When I first started on my recovery from Stroke I set the intention there and then that I would be able to walk The Ridgeway again. At that specific time, I couldn't hardly sit up in bed let alone walk "The Ridge", but I was determined, I set the intention six months before it eventually became a reality. We never know how long something may take to manifest into physical reality but as I've stated many times before, everything starts in the mind, the thought, the idea. That idea is fuelled by intention, emotional feelings and energy, and only then do we need to take aligned action to bring about the result into reality.

Transformation Key: If you want to manifest a new reality, start with the idea. Fuel the idea with intention, emotional feelings and energy and then take the aligned action to realise that reality.

119

25 March, 2022: It's Started

It's started!

As Claire, Toby dog and I walked into the woods this morning I called out to Claire, who was 20ft in front of me, "Look, they're starting to come out!"

I looked around, surveying the ground around us and there they were, new bluebells appearing for the 2022 season.

This initial showing will bloom into a magnificent carpet within 2 weeks.

I truly love this moment in the year as it defines one of the most beautiful moments of life in the woods. All the other phases of the year-round woodland cycle are in preparation for this coming dawn of purple haze. In 2 weeks we shall witness a natural splendour that is breathtaking and I am thrilled to bits with anticipation.

The cycle of life has so many moments of beauty and even in the seemingly dark days of winter the carefully choreographed sequence that is often hidden from view is carefully preparing the scene for the true moment of glory; the moment of the great revealing; the moment of complete oneness and perfect synchronicity that we shall all experience in time. The new will shine through; then move on to prepare the way for the next new; and so it goes on. For some, like myself, the moment of passing was not meant to be and the chance to witness such natural spectacles like the bluebells has been gifted to me once more.

Perhaps having come close to death has made the anticipation of this coming bluebell season all the more emotional and carries so much meaning.

After I'd taken photos I later stopped in my tracks as I listened to the combination of gentle piano music playing in my coat pocket mixed with the sound of birds in the woods. I was brought to tears in that instant; the emotional wave of pure gratitude washed over me. So utterly happy to be alive and witness that mix of complexity that landed with me so beautifully and simply in those couple of seconds.

What an experience this all is, I'm so lucky

To witness the bluebells in the local woods is a wonder of nature. It is breathtaking in its abundance.

Throughout the year the woods prepare the environment to produce the spectacular display that many local people enjoy.

It's amazing to see so many new faces enjoying the woods within that special period. It's a great shame that these same people don't get to witness the woods out of bluebell season for, in my opinion, the woods are just as magical.

But bluebell season is incredible and our family and I are blessed to have such a setting that yields this glorious display right on our doorstep.

This particular period of March 2022 was a sad time for my family. On March 23, 2022, my father passed on. He passed peacefully in hospital with choral music playing in his room. I was informed of his passing after it had actually occurred but I was the first of my three siblings to go to the hospital.

We were all expecting Dad to pass as his health and life force had deteriorated since November 2021, so his final passing was not a shock or surprise. I've always had a comfortable relationship with the thought of passing. To me, passing is a transition rather than a death. To me there is no death, there is only a transitioned state of being.

As I believe that our true nature is spiritual and energetic, then passing is a return to being whole again as that true nature. I truly believe that Dad is around and still with us, we just can't see him in the physical flesh.

I witness many signs of him being around, especially during that time in March. I recall seeing more Robins than usual, perhaps because it was springtime maybe, I don't know. I remember walking up to the woods and on the way there; on the track that leads to the woods, a Robin flew next to me almost all the way up the track, singing away to...something, maybe me, maybe not. Dad was a great singer so it was fitting that this Robin should accompany me in this way up to the woods. I remember calling out, " Hi Dad, I see you, I hear you." It was comforting if nothing else.

The bluebells and the cycle of the woods seemed to reflect my mindset with the cycle of life and the natural recycling of energy. It provided the perfect backdrop to process the passing of my Dad. The time that Claire and I spent at the log cabin, and the time I spent walking the Ridgeway, coupled with this time with the abundance of bluebells, all gave me precious time to listen to God within and to reflect and process the passing of my Dad. I feel the presence of Dad as I write this sat alone next to the sailing lake in late August 2022, he's always around.

Transformation Key: Nothing is forever. Everything is transient. Make the most of every moment.

120

〰️

1 April 2022: Neuropsychology Discharge

Neuropsychology Discharge.

Today, I received the official discharge letter from the Clinical Psychologist having been discharged in early March.

There are several areas that make me really pleased but mostly the fact that he cited the techniques and modalities that I have naturally adopted to support my own mental and emotional journey dealing with depression, anxiety and low mood. I recall his last conversation with me when he discharged me. He said, "The techniques you've developed yourself are as effective as anything I could offer. There's nothing more that I can offer."

During December 2021 I experienced depression, anxiety and suicidal ideation as a result of PTSD which I worked through myself and with the support of Claire. My clinical psychology sessions started in February 2022 (2 months later). By early January 2022, I was feeling far more upbeat and positive about the future. Today, I am flying pretty high with so much inner strength and self-assurance. The techniques that I've used include:

Journaling - writing things down is a wonderful way of expressing feelings and thoughts. I've been an over-thinker all my life and it's not healthy.

Spending Time Outdoors (Every Day) - the frequency of nature is right up there. Being in nature is perfection IMO. There's so much to relish and enjoy from our natural environment; it is a pure gift. Looking Forward whilst Savouring The Now - I'm an optimist, I always have been. I have a predominantly positive attitude and even when circumstances get challenging I (somehow) find the funny side or see the irony. I used to get so wrapped up in my past or the future whereas now I just enjoy "the now". Worrying (like I used to) about the past or the future is such a waste of energy; all I/we really have is now.

Gratitude - there's so much to be grateful for...the list is endless. Having cheated death 6+ months ago and having lived through depression and suicidal ideation, I am now so grateful to be alive.

Emotional Release - I remember permanently feeling an overwhelming sense of sadness in myself. I lived with that for years. Like many, I would mask it well and seem like a happy cheeky *chap but under the surface, I wasn't really happy. I recall having sadness rise within me but I could never cry. That has changed. I've allowed the tears to flow freely whenever they rise. Allowing the emotions to flow without any particular attachment or meaning is one of the best forms of release I have ever experienced. These techniques I developed and learnt from Claire. We don't claim to be clinical professionals but we are experienced at being the centre of trauma and the associated effects. No textbook can ever replace first-hand experience in any subject. Clinicians have their place, but I am living proof that you can do so much for yourself.*

Today I have great optimism for the future, whilst still revelling in the glory of now. One day I hope to help others on their own journey of recovery, healing and/or self-actualisation...although I recognise that this journey is never done...it is a continuous unfolding and discovery...wow what a journey life is!!!

This post from April 1, 2022, says it all.

Looking back at the transformation that was occurring is incredible. As I write this additional narrative in late August 2022, some 4/5 months later, I can say the transformation was permanent. It was life-changing. My recovery from Stroke and brain trauma is still ongoing but the transformation of my mindset feels permanent. My relationship with my God-self is established and ongoing. I am happy and content with life.

My journaling has turned into an enjoyment of writing. I love to write anything really. I'm enjoying the writing this book, I write for my job with marketing content creation, and I write small poems or inspired writing for blog posts in Stroke-related social media groups. The writing flows through and it's something that I love to share with others in the hope that I can inspire or offer hope for the future, especially those that have been affected by Stroke.

As previously written, the ability to spend time outdoors in nature is essential to my mental well-being and my ability to listen to God. Nature is the perfect antidote to our modern stress-ridden lives.

Overall the transformation of self that I have experienced more than anything has resulted in a deep feeling of contentment, love and satisfaction. I now revel in the present moment and don't get wrapped up in the torture of the mind judging the past or trying to control the future. After all, there is only now; this present moment. My gratitude for all aspects of life has grown exponentially through this inner work. I now don't feel the baggage of past trauma (PTSD) from emotional situations that I had previously labelled as bad, sad, hurtful, unfair, misunderstood or unworthy. The healing is predominantly done in that respect, but I know should anything arise again that I have the tools to release the emotion from my body forever.

Transformation Key: Develop the techniques that will serve you for life. They can save your life, transform your life and they are tools that will serve you and your loved ones forever.

121

10 April, 2022: Riding My Bike

Riding my bike.

Today I found the courage to start riding my bike again.

I tried riding it a few months or more back and it felt wrong; I was nervous; the anxiety kicked in; there was no logical reason for the nerves but nonetheless I felt weird.

I had set the intention to ride my bike yesterday but I ran out of time. So today I pumped up the tyres and set off.

I wasn't going far which is just as well because I could feel I was out of condition; the slopes felt like hills and the wind felt strong blowing against me.

I didn't care that the distance was small; I was not trying to set any records; I just wanted to get started.

That is the theme throughout my recovery from stroke. Just get started and do it!! Whatever it is, just do it!! Sometimes it's just not possible and that's ok; I've learnt how to be kind to myself and forgive myself when it doesn't feel right. But go back another day when so inspired.

Inspiration is that sense of hearing the inner voice that wants you to win. I sense that voice as the voice of God in those moments so it's time to take the inspired action; go and try and ride the bike again, it's time.

The good news is that I didn't fall off; I enjoyed the feeling of riding the bike again; I suppose a little like riding for the first time again; woohoo!

Do you remember those days as a child when making those first attempts at riding a bicycle? When I had originally tried earlier in my recovery it just didn't feel right and I lacked the confidence to continue. In those moments it's ok to 'step back' and not pursue the attempt. It's right to listen to that inner voice if (and only if) you know that voice is the voice of kindness and not the voice of fear.

At some point, that voice of kindness will suggest that it's time to try again. That voice of kindness and love, wants you to succeed, it wants you to overcome the fear and anxiety. That is the time to move and "do the thing".

That thing could be riding your bike again after a stroke (as in my case) or it might be that attempt at starting a new business, or trying a new sport, or walking in those shoes. It doesn't matter what the situation is, the point is about learning to listen to your inner voice and distinguishing your inner voice of love from your inner voice of fear.

The inner fear is from your ego mind whose sole purpose is to protect you. In doing so, that voice does serve a purpose so please don't think that that voice is in some way bad, it's not bad, it's just not always right.

The other inner voice of kindness and love is your God-self speaking to you. Your God-self has your best intentions at heart. It is pure love. It sounds like inspiration and appreciation of the present moment.

Your God voice is always trying to speak to you but so often it is drowned out by the noise of our human life on earth such as the noise from distractions, gossip, and fear-based conditioning. Only when we still our minds can we give our God-self voice a chance of filtering through.

Transformation Key: Only when we still our minds can we allow our God-self voice to filter through.

122

10 April, 2022: Happiness

I have been guilty of seeking happiness from external sources. Like so many, I used to seek happiness from:

Relationships

Cars

Bikes

Houses

Career

The next contract

Customers

...the list could be endless tbh

It has been through the inner work, guided with such skill and expertise by my future wife Claire, that I've come to realise that true happiness lies within and never without. True deep happiness can never be found in anything external (the without) but only in the inner relationship I have with myself.

We often hear the words 'you complete me' when referring to a loved one or spouse. When I think about that, it makes no sense at all. If we become dependent on anything external to 'compete us' then we are completely disempowered. When I became reunited with my inner being and started to have a compassionate conversation with that quiet part of myself, I then started to catch a sense of what happiness means. I felt empowered again.

I used to feel deeply unhappy despite the external 'things'. It was a horrible feeling. I could never figure out why. Since so much of my life was flipped on its head with the stroke, I've discovered so many nuances of myself that I had previously lost. Lost beneath layer after layer of programming, wounding, patterning and conditioning from the circumstances of life that can cause pain and emotional anguish which then meant reaching for the next 'thing'.

Since I've peeled back the layers and healed the emotional scarring I've come to the realisation that with the solidity of an inner heartfelt relationship with myself, there is the added benefit of the rediscovery of true happiness.

It is not a finished job by any means, but I do feel those moments of joy that I previously thought were lost and forgotten forever.

Say hello to your inner self and start a beautiful loving conversation - it will be the source of your true happiness.

To discover true happiness was one of the best gifts I could have ever been blessed with. For so long and an often default position of mine would be a gnawing sense of unhappiness within.

Like so many, I would seek happiness and relief from the unhappiness from external sources; TV, social media, shiny things like cars, motorbikes, houses and then more personal things like relationships, career progression, professional status and loved ones.

One of the aspects of my life that was deeply personal was the fear of losing my relationship with my youngest children following my marital breakup and divorce in 2014/2015. During the early months of my recovery, the financial situation was awful and that meant that I had to cut the voluntary child maintenance that I had been giving to my ex-wife.

Without going into the details, the thing that I came to realise was that I had voluntarily continued to pay out far above what was affordable because I feared that I would lose my relationship with my children. Losing the relationship with my children was one of my biggest fears and that fear had been killing me.

As a result of the stroke, being incapable of earning an income and having no income insurance meant that the maintenance had to be reduced and I had to seek the help of the Child Maintenance Service to establish what was affordable and realistic.

I knew that doing this would cause me to face one of my deepest fears. It also made me realise that in some way

I conditioned myself into thinking at a deep subconscious level that I was buying the love of my children. Of course, that kind of deep-rooted unconscious belief is a recipe for profound unhappiness.

When I faced my fears head-on and had no option but to take the plunge, I realised that my children loved me unconditionally. I already knew this in my logical, rational, conscious mind but in my subconscious mind and within my emotional body a different belief and pattern had been playing out for so long.

This is another example of the gift and awakening that has come with the stroke and I can pass it on to others, as my gift to share.

Being able to face fears head-on leads to life-long change, and in my particular case, being able to face deep-rooted fears, such as this actually led to a release from the grip of fear and that led to a discovery of a a greater feeling of happiness within.

I had let the fear control my mind, my behaviours and ultimately my happiness.

Transformation Key: When you stand up and face your fears, your fears then melt away right before your eyes; it was all make-believe in your mind. In that salvation can lie the source of true happiness.

123

12 April 2022: Yoga, Pilates, Strengthening, Gratitude

Yoga+Pilates+Strengthening+Gratitude.

Every morning after getting out of bed and every night before going to bed I do my exercise/physio. This is a "must" for me, not only for my continuous recovery but, just as importantly, for my ongoing mental, emotional and spiritual journey and transformation.

As I begin each "session" I always start by standing with my hands in prayer position and I give thanks and gratitude to The Universe/God for:

In the morning: The opportunity to experience another day on planet Earth and the beauty of the new day.

At night: The wonders of the day and all the amazing experiences I have been able to participate in.
I find these moments of intention and reflection serve me so well, they leave me fulfilled with a greater zest for life.

As mentioned before, I have developed my own version of a sun-salutation yoga flow routine that I have been doing morning and evening. Throughout the summer months, I dropped the evening routine as I simply enjoyed the late summer evenings walking the dog with Claire and, on occasion, the rest of the family.

The sun-salutation-based routine is predominantly based on yoga but I have also incorporated some of the pilates stretches that my physiotherapy team introduced me to, along with press-ups and tricep press-ups.

I supposed with all the elements put together into the continuous flow it probably takes me between 15 - 20 minutes to complete. I start by offering a prayer of gratitude and grounding into the new day giving thanks for the new day, my life and anything that comes to mind at the time, whether large or small. Nothing is deemed insignificant to give thanks to God for. Everything is equally 'important' in that sense. I can give gratitude for my life and my health as equally as I can give gratitude for the green grass within my view from the window.

I continue to hold the space for gratitude throughout the

flow routine so as to preserve that state of gratitude beyond the initial moment of prayer and reflection. As I move in the flow from pose to pose or stretch to stretch, I breathe in the light and love of divine consciousness and then equally I breathe out love and light to both consume the universal love and then give love back to the universe for the continual expansion of a loving universe. To me, this is a very personal spiritual experience as I exchange love energy and become very aware of my deep oneness and connection to everything and all potentialities.

Next time you perform your own yoga routine, whether it's an adaption similar to my own or a routine that is more aligned to a stricter discipline, try to engage at a deeper spiritual level that contributes to the loving expansion of the universe.

Transformation Key: Expand the universe with your loving energy and your life will become enriched with love and goodness.

124

14 April, 2022: Holding The Vision

Holding the vision.

Your thoughts create your reality, don't let your reality create your thoughts

Throughout my recovery from the debilitating effects of stroke, I have had to hold not just one vision but multiple visions of my desired future reality.

When I couldn't see, I had to re-imagine being able to see clearly again.

When I couldn't wash myself or get myself to the bathroom, I had to hold the vision of doing that again.

When I couldn't walk, I had to re-imagine walking steadily again.

When I couldn't talk, I had to imagine hearing my voice with clarity again.

When I couldn't work and earn any income, I had to hold the vision that one day that ability would return.... and so it goes on. When everything was stripped away from me in that fateful moment I had to learn how to create all over again. And what I learnt very quickly is this....

Everything is created from thought first...everything!

My/your/our reality is a projection of billions of simultaneous thoughts.

When I had nothing for that awful moment from the brain haemorrhage, I was actually handed a gift; it was an opportunity to start over.

My recovery is ongoing, I still feel a continuous sense of dizziness all the time but I know that one day that will stop. I know that because:

I imagine that and hold that vision.

and...

I take the actions aligned to that vision to support that vision coming into my reality.

This is it folks, the secret to your universe in one statement. Everything starts in the mind, literally everything. The power we all hold in our imaginations is unbelievable. So many of us have no idea of this power and often we create our realities by default. Sometimes that default turns out in our favour, whereas for others, or at a different period in life, that default can seem to kick us where it hurts. The crazy thing is, it is our own conscious and unconscious thoughts that start the entire process.

When I had a brain haemorrhage, I had to take a level of responsibility for that. I didn't consciously think to myself, "Oh I know, I think I'll have a brain haemorrhage, that's a good idea!" Of course not, that would be ridiculous and I'm not suggesting I consciously thought that, but did I subconsciously think thoughts on the same vibrational frequency as a brain haemorrhage? Well, the answer to that is probably yes. That may be unacceptable to some people and that's ok, not everyone will understand this way of thinking and that's ok, that doesn't mean anything right or wrong about me or them, it just is.

When I had a life (like many) led by egoistic governance the outcomes were not always going to be that favourable. When I say egoistic, I don't necessarily mean egoistic in the form of bragging, egoistic can equally mean a life based on fear, worry and living separated from self and oneness of all.

When I look back at my life pre-stroke it was predominantly based on fear and worry. I had some great experiences as well, but the underlying operating system was often run on anxiety, fear and control of the future. The stroke has made me realise that all we really have is now, this present moment. The past is just a series of memories and emotional impressions, and the future is simply projections in the mind of what we think the future might or might not be. So this means that all there actually is in this moment is now, and then now... and now, and now...

In fact, if we think about this even deeper, those moments make up our entire individual and collective versions of reality. It's like tiny snap-shots of now that are all strung together to make up the illusion of time...fascinating, don't you think?

125

18 April 2022: Field of Golden Carpets

Field of Golden Carpets.

As I walked Toby this morning I was struck by the beauty in everything. Not just the woods, which I've posted about plenty of times before, but also the golden carpets of dandelions in the fields.

They shine like miniature suns on the ground, radiating their golden yellow glow, almost lighting the way ahead.

Often overlooked and trodden upon, the dandelion is considered a weed by others (e.g. gardeners). When they tangle their way amongst a carefully curated flower bed they are an unwelcome intruder. But in the green fields of springtime, they hold their own, they stand out in their glorious majesty.

In that way, they symbolise and represent those that are often

> *overlooked and misunderstood. Everything and everyone has a place; all is beauty; all is an expression of divine intelligence or source energy.*
>
> *Let's hear it for "the dandelions"*

It's so easy to take things for granted. When I saw the dandelions that morning, I was struck by their radiance and the brightness that they seemed to shine out.

They were like little crowns of sunlight that carpeted the fields, lighting the way for the bees and butterflies. I believe some people pick them to make wine which I've never tasted and probably unlikely too since I'm now teetotal.

I made the decision to abstain completely from alcohol after I had a glass or two of Prosecco during the spring of 2022. The effect of the alcohol made me feel horrible and it reminded me of the awful effects of the brain haemorrhage during my early months of recovery. I thought, "Why the f... would I want to feel like that again? That's a stupid idea. No way, not for me thanks."

I don't judge others that like a drink but I've realised that I can go without it and I prefer the feeling of being clear-headed.

Claire and I went to a dance festival just a few days ago (September 11, 2022). We queued at one of the many bars on the huge site. I was looking to see if they had an alcohol-free lager on the menu, and yes, there was one listed 0% alcohol.

Perfect, I thought as I was expecting to purchase a soft drink loaded with sugar (another thing I'd rather avoid these days). Our turn arrived to be served and I asked for one of the 0% lagers. The server disappeared for a while and then returned with the news that they had all sold out. I had to have a sugary soft drink anyway! I found it interesting that of all the lagers, beers and ciders listed on the menu, it was the 0% alcohol one that had sold out. I suppose that shouldn't be a surprise for a dance festival where the common drink of choice is typically water, but I thought it was perhaps reflective of the times we now live in...maybe.

I think I was always ambivalent when it came to alcohol. It's never been a thing I've reached for as a means to obtain an alternative state of consciousness, in other words, I've never liked to get drunk. I've never been against drink or drinking as such but I have never been impressed by the effect that alcohol can have on people. I've witnessed some crazy situations and I'm sure we all know of some bad stories linked to alcohol and alcohol abuse. I used to enjoy a cider or a glass or two of red wine but if I'm honest with myself, it was always linked to some occasion, habitual situation or as a means to fit in with the circumstances.

Taking that self-awareness further, doing anything to fit in is always a judgement of self based on a lack of self-worth so perhaps the reason I drank (not to excess) in social situations was always linked to fitting in and a deep-rooted lack of self-worth that caused that need to fit in... that's interesting. Having a drink in a habitual situation is perhaps even more madness. I used to have a glass (or two, or three) after a week's work, almost like a reward of some kind. I'd use the excuse of wanting to relax and unwind after a stressful week. Really? Yes, I used to do that many years ago. Not surprisingly that habit soon resulted in weight gain. I stopped that routine as quickly as it started, but the crazy thing is, many people do that too. People drink alcohol as a means to dull the senses as part of a habitual regime, or because they think it's the thing to do in a social situation so they want to fit in. Why?

I don't now want to sound judgemental or self-righteous in any way. There's a saying that we use within our family, you do you and let me do me. If people want to drink that's fine by me as long it doesn't affect or do me any harm. I suppose all I invite others to consider is to ask themselves why are they having the drink, and then make a deliberate, conscious, and fully aware decision from that space rather than doing something just out of routine or habit, or from needing to fit in, that's all I'm saying.

Transformation Key: You do you, and let me do me. Don't ever feel pressured to do anything you don't want to do. You have your mind to make your own decisions.

126

18 April, 2022: Most Days...

Most days I feel a sense of how well my recovery has progressed.

I mean after 7 months after an almost fatal brain injury, I can perform most tasks pretty well (ish). That feels good and I am happy with the progress....I mean it's better than being dead or being in a permanent state of dependency, right? Of course it is, there's no question about that, and I'm eternally grateful for the chance to start over.

But there are moments in every day when I really notice my recovering brain. There are moments when I feel utterly sad and probably a bit sorry for myself if I'm honest with myself.

For a couple of hours today, I had that feeling. I had gone to do the grocery shopping, as I like to contribute towards the running of a busy family household. As I walked around the super-market trying to navigate people, shopping trolleys, the shopping list and trying to make decisions about items I couldn't find, I found myself slipping into a very low mood. I felt utterly pissed off about the whole shitty stroke situation.

I got home and Claire asked me what did I want to do this afternoon. I couldn't answer her. I felt paralysed and could not find any enthusiasm for anything. I wanted to be left alone.

My former self would have made this a thing. I might have made this feeling mean something about me in some way. I might have labelled it or judged myself for it. But these days I just take it for what it is...it's just energy...it's all just energy...and some-times that energy vibrates at a high frequency and sometimes at a lower frequency.

In moments like these, I just accept it. I witness it like a third party and most of all I don't make it mean anything at all.

It's all energy.

Acceptance and surrender are huge aspects of any recovery including my own. I am generally well known for my positive disposition and attitude towards life but there are times when that positivity can slip. In that way, I suppose, I am human. I might have achieved an incredible recovery but there are times when I can get down about the situation.

Every day as I walk around I will stagger or swerve if I'm

not careful. I will walk into things. My head feels foggy and I get muddled about situations. My memory is shockingly bad. I will forget words as I'm talking. I will forget why I've walked into a room or out of the room. I will completely miss out on words as I'm typing a sentence. I think the word is there but my fingers have not hit the keys to form the word and it's only after careful review that it will notice the glaring error. I notice the slight autism and perhaps others can see those traits too. I can only handle a maximum of two instructions at once. I cannot cope with complexity as I get too confused. Living with a brain injury and repairing the brain is not easy. Friends I spoke to about some of these traits will comment that they are like it too. For example, I was talking with a friend last week about my memory and about a situation where I had gone downstairs to do something or take something with me but when I got downstairs I had completely forgotten the thing from upstairs. I find this sort of thing frustrating so I have learnt to live with these things by laughing at myself and trying to not take the situation too seriously.

I suppose that is typical of me. If it were someone else who had the injury and these traits I would have compassion and I suppose the way I am compassionate with myself is to find humour within the situation. Maybe I'm just weird, I don't know, but it seems to work most of the time. That said, there are times when I get upset with myself. Perhaps a more accurate description is that I do feel the frustration and within that moment I haven't yet found the humour. When that occurs I can momentarily slip into a sadness about the brain injury. It would be very easy to get drawn into that sadness and feel sorry for myself, but I firmly believe that we get more of whatever we focus on. So using that logic, I refocus my attention, and therefore my energy, on humour and holding a vision of myself completely healed and fully recovered. If that strategy is still not working, I simply choose to think about something completely different and something that makes me happy and joyful.

Taking an immediate detour away from the current reality has been essential to my recovery so far and it is a strategy that I will continue to use throughout my life. "Get real!", is a phrase that people often use. Why do I want to get real? If I just focused on what was real then all I recreate in my life is that same version of reality; very much like the film Groundhog Day, where the lead character's life is repeated day after day until he makes a change. This is the same principle I have developed during my recovery. If I hadn't made a conscious decision to change something every moment of every day then I would still be stuck in that hospital bed.

Am I fully recovered yet? No, but I've come a long way in a relatively short time. All because of my unshakeable positive attitude towards life, fact!

Transformation Key: Develop an unshakeable positive attitude towards life for it will pay you huge dividends.

127

19 April, 2022: Another Day

Another day.

I taste the coffee. It's aroma fills my senses. The caffeine enters my body as I look out at a lone deer in the distance. The deer is gently grazing but ready to run at any time. The sun lights the fields and distant woodland.

What a blessing I am gifted with in this moment.

My initial sense of loss and grief for my old self is quickly replaced with a sense of gratitude for the new version of me; this is Me v.3

V1 was born and grew up innocent in the countryside. He took on some wounds that would remain with him for a long time. I love v1 for he was just a little boy trying to find his way in a strange world. V1 knew the truth; he was a creator with divine energy in his heart. He knew it and tried to express it as best he could but he ultimately felt like he didn't fit it. But he knew he was as unique as the next person; all unique but all connected as onenesses. "What is this?", he would think to himself. "Am I God?" Don't be daft came back the ego-based answer, "Who do you think you are?" But in his heart, he knew there was a truth to that question. V2 grew into a man but he buried his truth. He had let the ego self of worry, fear and doubt take centre stage. He was the provider and had to prove himself worthy of that title. This took him on a path that was not really him; not his true self that lived in his heart and soul. My divine self tried to make himself heard but my ego self was scared and didn't want to listen. Ultimately, v2 had to go. He was a good bloke but the operating system was based on fear and worry. On Sept 11, 2021, Me v2 was retired and decommissioned...a massive reboot was started.

And so Me v3 was birthed. He had to start over. Everything was shifted and turned over. Imagine all aspects of life are carefully placed upright in a box and then someone turns the box on its side. The entire contents fall into a heap. Even my vision was turned on its side for a while. Life was smashed and in pieces. Certain parts remained intact and helped me establish v3. So v3 was born and is still a work in progress. I am a creator and I create with my thoughts. I always have been, it's just that I've just remembered. I have rediscovered my soul and connection with my divine self. Me v3 can be anything I choose.

No version was/is good or bad, it was all part of the journey; all

> *part of the experience and I am blessed today that the experience*
> *goes on for another day.*

This post fully reflects the awakening and transformation that was taking place. As depicted within the post, I think of myself as different versions of the same human. All of these versions are me and I love them all equally. Like an evolving software package or computer operating system, each version builds upon the last, and like some operating systems, some versions might have more bugs and glitches than others, and each new version comes with a bunch of new features and enhancements.

Imagine looking through the features list and known bugs list of the different versions of yourself. What would you read?

So Me v3 had been created on that fateful day of September 11, 2021. When I think back to that day and the earlier parts of that day, I realise that I can't remember a lot of it. Was that because I was living in a daydream? Perhaps. I know I was completely unaware of what was about to occur in my life. Unprepared is probably a better description. But that is probably a good thing I think. If I had known ahead of time what was about to occur, what then?

Continuing on the operating system metaphor, if I were to return to pre-stroke life I would have to possess a complete system backup which would then be fully restored. Well, thankfully that is not possible. There is no backup and restore functionality for humans. We are evolving creatures, always changing, always transforming, always growing, always expanding, always unfolding in every moment. Thank God there is no going back!

I'm sure some people might think I'm slightly mad by saying that and perhaps that would have been the opinion of my former v2 self. That is completely understandable. No one in there right mind would raise their hand to volunteer for stroke or queue up to say "Oh yes please, I'll have one of those brain haemorrhages, they sound great fun!" Of course not, but when that situation occurred with all of the resulting awakening and transformation I look at it all now and say wow, maybe that was all for me, and none of it happened to me. Thinking that the stroke happened to me is a very victim-mode mentality which in itself is very debilitating and destructive, whereas when I think about the stroke happening for me, the mentality switches to one of empowerment, expansion and enrichment. Again, some people might struggle to understand this thinking and might well disagree, and that is ok with me, we don't all have to agree with my views on this, but taking this view has provided me with, what I can only describe as, spiritual fuel for my recovery.

Transformation Key: Nothing happens to you, it all happens for you at some level. Taking this view will give you the spiritual fuel to recover, heal, learn and grow.

128

❦

20 April, 2022: The Inner Voices

The inner voices.

Have you ever stopped to notice the constant and ongoing narrative going on in our heads? That narrative is either one of love or one of doubt, but nonetheless, the narrative is always there.

I have always been aware of the inner conversations I have with myself; perhaps this is something that other people are not aware of, but it is definitely something I have tuned into all my life. I've never spoken about it before for fear of being labelled a schizophrenic but these are not voices in my head that are urging me to hurt anyone or cause any harm to anyone, but nonetheless there are two types of conversation going on.

When people are truly honest and authentic they actually admit and realise that these two types of inner voice exist. The voice of *love and then the voice of doubt.*

The voice of love, well guess what, it loves us; your inner-self of love, well it loves you, it's as straightforward as that. It's always there if we tune into it. It's a love of kindness and self-care and a voice of new ideas and creative action of an expansive nature which creates even more love in the ever-expanding universe of spiritual mind. The voice of love is your own personal cheerleader willing you onward when the going gets tough or when the odds seem impossible and everything is stacked against you; even the doubt of others. The voice of doubt is the opposite. It wants to highlight our separateness from one another. It feeds upon our fears and it limits our expansion. It wants us to stay small. It would prefer that we stay locked away in our self-made prisons in the mind. Its function is to protect us and experience the world in such a way that pure love cannot. In that experiential way, it serves a great purpose, but if left unchecked it has incredible power to extinguish the voice of love if we allow it.

In that way, we have a choice. We are always at choice. In any given moment (now, now, now, now...) we can choose our thoughts and those thoughts create images in the mind and the voices we hear (again in the mind). We can choose which voice to listen to; both are present all the time.

I've learnt some massive lessons during my continuous recovery and transformation, and BTW there is no end to transformation, not for me and not for you (well not until we inevitably die that is and we pass onto the next dimension).

With the transformation of recovery, I've had to tame the voice of doubt and focus on the voice of love.

There is no concept of only one and not the other. They are neither good nor bad, they just are. Both are gifts and both are necessary, the only question is, which one will dominate? Love or Doubt?

With love

So which voice is the dominant one? The inner voice of love, compassion, kindness and possibility, or the voice of doubt, worry, fear, and conflict?

We get to experience both often dependent on the circumstances, but when we let the voice of doubt and fear dominate then we are more likely to navigate the world in an egoistic state and live in perpetual separateness.

The state of separateness occurs because the ego mind has taken over, and in doing so, we often block out the subtler voice of love. The voice of love is quieter and softer. We feel that voice rather than hear it in the mind. The feeling of love, compassion, kindness and possibility is felt in the body, like the heart or the gut, and it is intuitive and can sometimes be the quietest of whispers.

We tend to allow ourselves to be bombarded with noise linked to the voice of doubt which of course can make matters even worse. Now the voice of doubt is often not even our voice, but the voice(s) of external-based source(s). We have to become mindful of what we tune into and what we allow into our modes of reception via our senses of sight, hearing, smell, taste and touch, with the predominant senses being sight and hearing. We are receiving information all the time and we are then interpreting everything through our brains and neurology based upon patterns, recognition, biases and familiarity. We unconsciously seek out information that supports our current worldview and beliefs. If that worldview is based on our voice of fear and doubt then that's what we find more of in the world, more fear and more doubt. Conversely, if we've allowed the voice of love and kindness to dominate then we unconsciously find evidence to support that belief and pattern. I know very clearly which I prefer.

Transformation Key: Let your inner voice of love and kindness dominate your existence then you will find more evidence to support that loving worldview.

129

22 April, 2022: Going Strong

Going Strong.

This morning I was discharged by another clinical team (I think that's all of them now!!)

I had a repeat visit to the Eye Clinic at 8:15 a.m. and by 9:00 we were finished. Sandra, the clinician said, "Ok, everything is great, I'm going to discharge you, I don't need to see you again." She then added that when she looked at my notes from my CT scan taken on 24 Dec 2021 (the date of my relapse) the CT scan showed that the original haemorrhage had fully recovered (aka totally gone/healed up/disappeared).

Holy F that was the best news ever!!

No one had told me that....errrr did they not think that might be important?! Anyway, whatever, communication is not the strongest point of the NHS So a double whammy of goodness for me this morning.

As I contemplate this again as I go to bed, I have to say I'm pretty damn pleased, to say the least

And the news yesterday that I can share my story to help many others via a cool new App featuring my story in film, I can say that these last few days have been amazing.

...and I also got to see my Mum today for the first time since October last year. Today was her 87th birthday, so Claire and I went to visit today which made her super happy.

More please Universe.

There was so much to celebrate on April 22, 2022, (that's a lot of 2's, I like that!) Mum's birthday, getting officially discharged from the Orthoptic Department of the hospital with a clean bill of health for my eyesight and then hearing the news that during my CT scan on Dec 24, 2021, the brain haemorrhage was found to be completely resolved. I had no idea what that even meant. Resolved? Why is it that specialists speak in technical ways? And didn't anyone think to inform me? Clearly not, but on April 22, 2022, I didn't care about that. Although the news was almost 4 months late, I was delighted. Although I understood from my research that the brain tissue within the affected area had died, the fact that my body had cleared up the blood in that area still meant that my brain and body were naturally doing what was correct, the body had cleared up then blood and my brain was busy rebuilding the missing neurology.

Transformation Key: Trust in the process. There will be times when you cannot see the results of your efforts, but through trust, persistence and faith you will get there.

130

29 April, 2022: Pathways

Pathways.

You may well ask what have these images got to do with neural pathways and brain function?

Let me explain...

It hit me today as I walked around the woods, how the blockages in the woods are representative of the damage that can be caused to the brain as a result of a stroke.

A fallen tree or branch will block the normal route taken by humans or animals and this is very much like the effect on the brain from stroke. The normal and established path is blocked.

But the amazing thing is that new pathways are formed in order to continue the route. This is exactly the same for the brain...new pathways are established in order to continue the journey and reach the destination.

I love thinking of weird sh!t like this!!

The woods where I walk every day near my home are a perfect metaphor for the rebuilding of neural pathways in the brain after damage has occurred.

As I walk around the woods I see branches and even whole trees that have fallen and that now block a former route and pathway that had been long established. The route may have been created by animals or humans that roam and walk the woods but now with the blockage in the way a new route needs to be established. As before, most of these new pathways are started by animals and then human walkers will typically follow suit and thus a new route is eventually formed.

This is exactly like the brain and the damage that can occur within neurology. When damage occurs, new neurology must be formed. Just like an alternative pathway through the woods because of a fallen tree.

I first pondered this metaphor when one of the visiting physiotherapy team Kate told me what happens with brain damage. I recall thinking about the idea of travelling from my nearest town, Swindon, to London via the M4 and then imagining that the M4 was then closed and a new route had to be established across fields, streams, ditches and hedges. In my imagination, I pondered the difficulties of such a task. Needless to say for the first travellers to establish the new route the journey would be difficult, and tiring and those initial travellers could easily be tempted to give up at any point. But as more and more travellers used the same route, then the journey would become slightly easier with each completed journey.

This is the same for the brain. Initially, the journey of neural connectivity and communication and therefore the ability for a message to correctly reach its destination is difficult. Over time and continual use (i.e. repetition) neurology becomes ingrained and reliable. Eventually, the pathway is so defined that neurological brain responses become automatic.

We take the complexities of our brains for granted. It was only as a result of sustaining damage to my brain that I became acutely aware of the complexities that were taking place. Consider some of the mundane activities that we often do and imagine all of the neural messages passing around the brain so fast to complete those activities.

Imagine you want to make yourself a cup of caramel latte coffee from a coffee pod machine. This sounds like a straight-forward task, right? No, it's not and yet it's something that I, and millions of others in the world, probably do every day without much conscious thought. Every action is under-taken based on the instructions and patterns that we have established within our brains and our subconscious minds. Think about every action and break it all down into each task and subtask, the list is almost endless. Well, each one of those tasks involves neural communication within the brain, and each piece of communication has to be transmitted and received in the right way, in the right order, the electrical signal, and the release of the correct hormone and chemical has to occur at the right time in the right quantity which then stimulates the muscles and tendons to carry out the correct physical movement to carry out the task. Then each task provides feedback through the senses which has to be processed so that we can make sense of the task currently taking place, and all of this happens at the same time we might be making our breakfast, listening to the radio, watching TV, looking at our smartphone, as well as a million other tasks controlling our breathing, our heart, our blood pressure, all of the receptors linked to our senses, and more and more. All require our neurology to work exactly as intended so that we don't forget the coffee or spill it all over the floor.

Don't you agree, that you and I are amazing creatures?

Transformation Key: You are the most amazing creature and you are gifted with an incredible brain. Don't ever take that gift for granted.

131

30 April 2022: Massive Proud Moment

> *Massive proud moment!!!*
> *My boy got picked to play for the Wessex Warriors U13s cadet rugby 7's side and has been playing at Twickenham today!!*
> *He's missing his regular club teammates who are on tour this weekend but playing at the English home of rugby is going to be a lifelong memory!*
> *I'm so proud of him and chuffed for him.*

As you've been reading this book, you may have figured out the significant part that rugby has placed within this story. The fact that the brain haemorrhage happened while volunteering at the local rugby festival, then being able to watch my son train and take part in matches during my recovery and being able to walk back into the clubhouse. Rugby has punctuated the story and recovery.

So it was fitting to add this post and diary entry too. My recovery was strong enough to enable Claire, Charlotte, Roger and I to attend the famous annual Army vs. Navy fixture at the home of English Rugby, Twickenham Stadium in southwest London. What made that event even more special was to be able to witness my son playing for an army cadets team representing the southwest region of England. He played several games and even played during the half-time break of the men's fixture in front of over 58,000 people. What an honour for him and all of us in attendance.

We had tickets for seats high up in the upper tier of the stadium so it was almost impossible to pick out my son from that distance but knowing he was there and that I had got there to witness it was a huge event.

Transformation Key: Trust that God will provide for you in ways far greater than you can ever imagine.

132

7 May, 2022: Closure

Closure.

Today was the day that I found closure to the major trauma I experienced on Sept 11, 2021, the day I experienced a cerebral haemorrhage.

Like a time bomb, it struck without any warning or consideration. Causing such an immediate and lasting impact.

The last 8 months have tested my resolve to the very limit; I've discovered a new version of me which was the gift I decided to take from a potentially devastating scenario. I've learned to accept and forgive my new self for daily mishaps whilst recovering from brain trauma. I've learned to accept the loss of my old self whilst rediscovering aspects of my personality that used to stay hidden out of fear or doubt. I now understand the meaning of that day.

Today I volunteered at the local rugby club (RWBRFC) cider and sausage festival. It was a day of mixed emotions and the sights and smells as I walked into the beer tent triggered memories of brain trauma that were rooted in my body. There were moments when I questioned what was I doing. But my determination overruled any anxiety or concern. ...and what a day it was. I met people who had tried to help me but like everyone else who witnessed me on that day, they thought I was drunk, not suffering a brain haemorrhage!!! The specific man in mind kept returning to talk to me today. My story triggered his own childhood memories of his grandfather who had been affected by stroke. He was amazed to be having a conversation with me. Statistically, I should have died.

So the day is done! I have experienced closure on the whole life-changing experience.

There is no closure to the effects that continue to this day. But to relive the moments in such detail was a huge step today and one I am pleased to say passed without any drama at all :-)

So this was the day that I could finally put the trauma of September 11, 2021, to rest and get some form of mental closure. Returning to another event exactly like I had been at when the brain haemorrhage occurred; the same place, the same beer tent, the same smells, surrounded by the same people, and similar sounds was a chance to truly face the fears of the past. Whilst I still feel the effects to this day, the anguish and trauma of the event have passed.

The trauma that my body had experienced just 8 months

earlier had been life-changing. I had experienced nothing like I could have ever imagined so to be able to almost re-live the moment felt surreal.

Was I anxious? You bet!

When I walked into the beer tent, the actual place where it all initially happened, I must admit the smell of the BBQ, cooked burgers and the sight of the barrels of beer and cider, nearly made me vomit. I nearly turned back and walked back out unable to fulfil my intention of capturing the moment with some pictures.

Alfie was there, just like before when we had been serving together. Claire got a picture of us together and then that was enough for me, I had to get out of there.

I didn't get to serve cider with Alfie again but it felt good to be able to exorcise the fears and "demons" from my body.

Claire and I then got into volunteer mode for the rest of the day and sold tokens for the beer/cider and BBQ. Claire ran the money, whilst I organised the tokens into batches of 10 to make the process of selling and distributing them easier. We make a great team!

The day passed without a hitch and I met one of the guys (John) who had been near the van when I had been escorted there by Claire on that fateful day in September 2021. John had said that he would keep an eye on me whilst Claire had returned to her duties on the BBQ and rounded up all the kids. When we met him again 8 months later, he started chatting to us and then Claire told him what had happened to me. His jaw visibly dropped to the floor. He hugged me and couldn't believe what he was hearing. John returned several times during the afternoon. He told me his own story linked to a stroke. He kept repeating himself about how it was incredible that I was standing in front of him now, alive and kicking. Like many others, he admitted that when he saw me he just thought that I couldn't handle my drink and would wake up the following morning with a hangover from hell. Er, hell, yes, hangover, no.

Transformation Key: People will be shocked at your transformation and many will want to celebrate you.

My Yoga Poses (Asana) Flow and Strength Training Routine

This flow was adapted by me from several sun salutation flows that I have participated in during numerous yoga classes that I attended in the past. I also added some Pilates and strength training routines as well. I practice this routine twice a day (morning and night). This flow is developed to be completed twice in a single practice (first on the left side and then on the right side). The first round will have the first Lower Lunge with Prayer starting on the left leg (ie. the left leg is back with the right leg forwards at a 90-degree angle at the knee). After the Downward Facing Dog, the second Lower Lunge is then performed by taking the left foot forward between the hands with the right leg back before flowing into the Warrior 2 which will be performed with the left foot forward and the right left back. The Warrior 2 then flows into the Resolved Triangle which again in the first round has the left foot forward and the right foot back. The final Lower Lunge with Prayer flows out of the Revolved Triangle and once again, continues with the left foot forwards and the right foot back. Upon completion (with Mountain with Prayer Hands) of the first round (left side), I then continue with the right side focus as I start the flow again from the top (Standing Backbend (back) with Prayer Hands).

English Name	Sanskrit Name
Standing Backbend (back) with Prayer Hands	
Standing Forward Bend	Uttanasana
Mountain with Prayer Hands	Tadasana
Chair with Prayer Hands	Utkatasana
Lower Lunge with Prayer Hands (1st)	Anjaneyanasa
Plank	
Four-limbed Staff	Chaturanga Dandasana
Tricep Press-up x 10	
Upward facing dog (cobra)	Urdhva Mukha Svanasana
Downward facing dog	Adho Mukha Svanasana
Lower Lunge	Anjaneyanasa
Warrior 2	Virabhadrasana 2
Revolved Triangle	Parivrtta Trikonasana

Lower Lunge with Prayer Hands (3rd)	Anjaneyanasa
Chair with Prayer Hands	Utkatasana
Mountain with Prayer Hands	Tadasana

After I've regained my breath, I then move into a Press-up position and do 50 press-ups.   The Press-ups do tire me and I will be out of breath after completion so I then move into the final part of my routine which is a combination of Child pose followed by a series of Cat and Cow based postures.

Childs Pose	Balasana
Cow x 10	Bitilasana
Cat x 10	Marjaryasana

The Cat/Cow poses alternate one to the other Cat, Cow, Cat, Cow and I do each Cat/Cow combination 10 times.

Almost there - The next part of my routine is to stay on all fours and then (alternating right side then left side), I reach up and then reach through to twist my core 10 times (each side).

Finally, I finish with 10 x Opposition Reach; extending my left arm out front whilst simultaneously extending my right leg out towards the back. Switch to do 10 x Opposition Reach again, but this time extending the right arm out front whilst simultaneously extending the left leg towards to back. Throughout these twenty reps, I maintain a strong straight spine during the extension and squeeze my stomach muscles on the contraction before turning to the extensions.

Finished!

My Blood Pressure Results

Monitoring my blood pressure has become a critical component of my life. Whilst I have learned to not let any given result define my mental well-being, it is still, nonetheless, essential for my physical well-being. Through carefully controlled medication and management of stress, I have successfully brought my blood pressure to a stable state. The results shown below show monthly averages between September 2021 and September 2022.

Monthly Averages			
Month	**Systolic**	**Diastolic**	**Range**
Sep '21	153	96	High Blood Pressure (Hypertension) Stage 1
Oct '21	150	100	High Blood Pressure (Hypertension) Stage 1
Nov '21	135	89	Prehypertension
Dec '21	130	86	Prehypertension
Jan '22	133	84	Prehypertension
Feb '22	126	85	Prehypertension
Mar '22	137	85	Prehypertension
Apr '22	138	86	Prehypertension
May '22	132	88	Prehypertension
Jun '22	124	83	Prehypertension
Jul '22	114	77	Normal
Aug '22	116	77	Normal
Sep '22	114	76	Normal

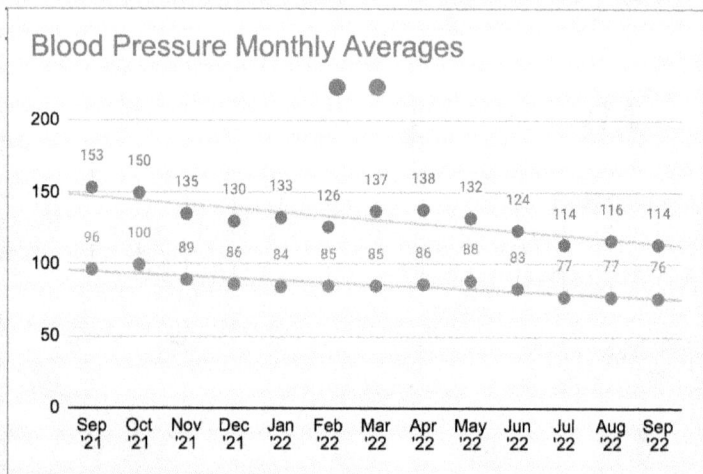

Blood Pressure Monthly Averages

The End - Afterword

So that's the end of this book but the recovery continues to this day and perhaps for the remainder of my life and I've accepted that; I'm at peace with that; I've accepted who I am and who I am becoming. I live with the effects of brain trauma every day (unbalanced, forgetfulness, etc.) and I have learned to embrace my life with absolute gratitude for every moment I have. My ability to work has been impacted due to my preference to only work remotely due to an increased level of anxiety about unfamiliar and stressful situations; that preference is born out of my prioritisation for my physical, mental, emotional and spiritual well-being. This impacts my ability to earn a living like I used to and I'm thrilled to be creating a new career as an author as well as a transformation consultant and coach.

There are moments when the future might concern me, but being concerned is just a form of fear, and fear stands for False Evidence Appearing Real. Who knows what the future holds? What is this concept we call the future anyway? Even my rational mind can understand that the future is merely a projection of my own thoughts. All we truly have is this

explosive moment of creation that happens now, now, now...
Our past is a collection of memories and the future is a collection of ideas and thoughts. I do know that holding the
vision of what I desire and feeling into what those desires
will yield in the form of emotions will bring forth those
desires. When I couple those thoughts and feelings with
taking aligned action whilst deeply appreciating the present
moment, I know it will ultimately yield an amazing outcome.
So all those false illusions wrapped up as fear of the future
can jump in the back seat of the car for the ride, as I choose
to sit in the driving seat, take the wheel and allow all the
goodness to flow to me.

"The Gift" is a message of hope. Hope not only for me but for
everyone. It is so easy to become immersed in the challenges
that life can seemingly throw at us. Those struggles can appear
to be so real in the moment, but when we look beyond any
trial, we come to recognise that life is not out to "get us".
We are powerful creators who can assert our own will on the
direction of our lives. When we are reminded of this, we are
given hope.

The lessons I've learned from this experience are extensive,
but there are things I think we all know for sure, but many of
us forget, so here are 10 top tips worth remembering:

1. Life is a journey of continuous change: it's an over-used
   cliche but it's fundamentally true, and we never know
   what's around the corner. Embrace change.

2. We will all leave this earthly realm at some point and there is nothing to be afraid of.

3. We are primarily spiritual and pure energy in nature and this physical experience on planet Earth is merely transitory but while we're here let's make the most of it. It's an amazing playground in which to revel and create.

4. We are here to learn and expand. There is a lesson in everything.

5. We are here to help one another (thanks for this one Dad).

6. We are always at choice in how we think and therefore feel, so use your thoughts wisely. Your thoughts and feelings really do create your reality.

7. Even if we're having a rough time, the time will eventually pass and we'll experience something else. Be open to learning the lesson and welcome the next unfolding; remember change is constant.

8. We are blessed to have this experience called life so don't waste it.

9. Our brains are incredible so look after yours; it's so precious.

10. Love one another, and be kind and compassionate with all living things.

Simon

www.ingramcontent.com/pod-product-compliance
Lightning Source LLC
Chambersburg PA
CBHW051707020426
42333CB00014B/878